For Chak and Cath
with love
from
B. & T.

December 1991

SNAPSHOTS IN TIME

Some experiences in health care
1936 - 1991

Chairman: Cornwall & Isles of Scilly AHA, 1967-77
Chairman: Paddington & North Kensington HA, 1981-86
Chairman: Kensington, Chelsea & Westminster FPC, 1979-85
Member: Medical Research Council, 1979-87
Member: Lambeth, Southwark & Lewisham FPC, 1987-90
Vice Chairman: Lambeth, Southwark & Lewisham FHSA, 1990-
Vice Chairman: (formerly Director), Disabled Living Foundation, 1981-

by Belinda Banham

with an introduction by Sir Patrick Nairne

The Patten Press
Newmill 1991

Published for The Jamieson Library of Women's History by The Patten Press, The Old Post Office, Newmill, Penzance, Cornwall TR20 4XN.

First issued in this paperback edition 1991

ISBN 1 872229 01 8
Jacket design: Carole Page
Photographic work: Bob Berry
Printed in Great Britain by Billing & Sons, Worcester.

Table of contents

FOREWORD

When in Autumn, 1975, I arrived at the Elephant and Castle, as a permanent secretary new to the Department and a stranger to the National Health Service (NHS), I was soon introduced to Belinda Banham as one of the most experienced 'Chairs' in the Service. She had had then some 40 years of service - from nursing on the wards of a Margate Tuberculosis hospital to chairing the Cornwall and Isles of Scilly Area Health Authority - and further advancement lay ahead.

In 1977 a career that had taken her from the bedside to the boardroom widened into fresh, and even more exacting, fields. In that year she became Director of the Disabled Living Foundation, a year later a member of the Medical Research Council, and in 1981 Chair of Paddington and North Kensington Health Authority - only four years after she had resigned from the Cornish chair with the well-deserved honour of the C.B.E. As if that was not enough, she was also by then Chair of the Kensington, Chelsea and Westminster Family Practitioner Committee (FPC). And now in 1991, with those appointments behind her, she is still at work in the NHS as a member of another FPC, now called the Family Health

ςℓℓvices Authority (FHSA), serving Lambeth, Southwark and Lewisham.

This remarkable book, SNAPSHOTS IN TIME,
tells her story of over 50 tireless years devoted to
the care and welfare of the sick, the handicapped,
the disturbed, and the homeless. It is not, as she
explains, an autobiography; but, while the private
person remains hidden, the character of a capable
and courageous public servant emerges clearly.
Nor is it, as she also makes clear, a history of the
NHS, though the incidents she describes vividly
convey the extraordinary evolution of a 'cottage
industry' service into the 'high tech' and
'unionised' NHS of today - with the consequent
and inescapable tension between expectations
and resources. It will be a useful source for the
historian of the Service.

Her 'snapshot' chapters, covering the different
phases of her career and her varied fields of responsibility, reveal why Belinda Banham always
found new doors being opened to her. She could
draw on wide practical experience of problems on
the spot, her mind was never shut to new ideas,
and she always remained ready to learn, not least
from her own mistakes.

Nothing shows her to better advantage than her
own confession in Chapter 13 that, experienced

though she was, her judgement could be wrong: "In those months of unrest," she wrote of her experience as Chair of Paddington and North Kensington in the 1980s, "I made several serious errors of judgement which could have had serious consequences..." They were 'errors' which reflected her characteristic determination to face a threatening challenge, and from the testing strains of an inner city health authority during the last decade she emerges with considerable credit.

So she does from the writing of this book - an achievement which other NHS Chairs have not matched. The book is a contribution to social history, a testimony to the quality of commitment which many women and men bring to the NHS; and a personal story which the countless friends and admirers of Belinda will enjoy.

Patrick Nairne

PREFACE AND ACKNOWLEDGEMENTS

This is not a history of the National Health Service nor of the hospitals in which I worked or for which, in later years, I bore some responsibility. Neither is this an autobiographical account of the whole of my professional life. Some episodes have been omitted, participants or their families remaining alive and being vulnerable to hurt by remembrance. Rather, this is my attempt to respond to requests to set down for posterity some sketches or snapshots of health care services as I perceived and experienced them over a period of momentous change and unprecedented challenge.

Tribute is due to so many for their support over these years, and I hope that my 'snapshots' will make this fact and my gratitude clear. More especially I dedicate this 'album' to Andy, the late Leslie, Joe and David, whose wisdom and counsel as Vice Chairmen was beyond price. I have also written it for John, Alan, Terry and Barbara, for the many staff whose loyalty and friendship made achievements in health care and services possible, and for my husband without whose encouragement and support I could not have persevered. Grateful thanks are due to my Secretary Mrs. Gwen Hill who worked with me in Cornwall, and whose unremitting patience and enthusiasm in the course of drafting and redrafting this book from many pages of manuscript was far beyond the call of duty.

Chapter 1
Early diagnosis and prognosis

The opening sequences of any life are shrouded in the mists of childhood memories. I was an only child, orphaned by death and the result of war. Nurtured on Victorian novels - the central theme of which often was prolonged wasting illness and death - together with an avid reading of A.J. Cronin's stories, of Vera Brittain's *Testament of Youth,* and of the heroism of Edith Cavell, my imagination was readily fired with a desire to emulate those heros and heroines of fact and fiction.

During the formative years of childhood and early adolescence an inspiring guide and mentor was to be found in our family doctor, James Falconer of Brixham, a man of great wisdom and compassion and the embodiment of all that was best in medicine in the years between the wars. Through him I gained access to the small cottage hospital which served our locality. In that place a surprising variety of procedures were undertaken which today would be regarded as totally unacceptable. But, this was not my only avenue by which I could enter vicariously the world of medicine.

From the window of the dormitory I shared with four others at boarding school - standing on an upturned locker, with the help of powerful binoculars - I could have a view of surgery being undertaken in a small hospital one field away. The frosted window of the operating theatre, extending only part way up, allowed excellent vision of the first incision but no clear sight of abdominal contents. Final closure could be clearly seen, as could other procedures such as wound cleansing after road traffic accidents - markedly less frequent than today - and sporting injuries and other trauma. I was a devoted one person gallery.

As school leaving time approached, the possibility and indeed the likelihood of a second World War dominated our thinking. Such thoughts reinforced my determination to enter medicine. Thus, I argued, whether through sentiment or cowardice, I would never be asked to take life, but would be trained and qualified to attempt to succour and maybe save. Though the time was still far distant when girls automatically looked toward a career, my determination was treated with kindly tolerance in the family and even encouraged, with the proviso that I could not enter medicine before attaining majority. At that age I would inherit sufficient money to supplement any scholarship I might gain for University.

With University entrance and the right subjects to gain exemptions from First MB, I was despatched, at age sixteen,to Brussels to gain a little culture. I should acquire fluent French, passable German and Italian, and in short, to 'finish' my general education. Within hours of arrival, I discovered the Edith Cavell Clinic located close by the school. Rapidly I migrated from the school to the clinic, ostensibly to help the nuns in caring for the patients.

The Royal Sea Bathing Hospital, Margate
1935-1937

On returning to England, the thought of waiting for four years to start a medical education proved intolerable. By dint of a slight bending of the rules over minimum age of entry, I began my training as a nurse in a special hospital for surgical and other tuberculosis. Due to my age I was limited to working on the children's wards but within six months this restriction was lifted. Life began in earnest.

The Royal Sea Bathing Hospital at Margate is situated on the sea front with only an esplanade between the wards and the sea. In the late 1930s the care and treatment of those suffering from orthopaedic and other forms of tuberculosis consisted, for the most part, in exposure to the elements. This exposure was certainly an adjunct to the very radical surgical procedures practised since drug therapy was not yet established. The wards were Nightingale in design, each giving on to two verandahs, one on either side. The verandahs were equipped with shutters which were never to be closed in the day, and at night only with permission of the night sister. Permission was seldom granted even when snow was falling, as it was thought contrary to the patients' interests. Cloaks were allowed to nurses only in moving to and from the wards. Strength and stamina were prerequisite to survival.

The majority of surgical tuberculosis patients required daily or twice daily dressings as wounds discharged profusely. These dressings were carried out at the bedside following a strict routine of techniques. Sterilisation of instruments, bowls and kidney dishes was by boiling. Dressing material was packed in drums, the dressings having been cut and folded, and wool rolled by nurses during the night. The drums were packed and transported to the autoclaves by nursing staff. They were responsible for autoclaving and for confirming sterility by the use of 'witness tubes.'*

It is difficult today to conceive of the patience and heroism of the patients occupying those beds. The

*   Chemical in small glass tube placed in centre of autoclave drum to 'witness' temperature change in sterilisation.

length of stay was indeterminate and never less than six months even in minor cases. With tuberculosis of the spine, frequently accompanied by psoas abscess, two or three years was common.

"Incise a tuberculous abscess and you sign that patient's death warrant" was a principle constantly taught. The result of ignorance or ignoring that dictum was frequently demonstrated by the onset of fatal amyloid disease or amyloidosis.

Surgery was as heroic as the patients who submitted to it. Amputation under local anaesthesia, excision of the head of the femur, and other major procedures were undertaken without the back-up of readily available blood and with no antibiotic cover or other modern adjuncts. Despite such disadvantages, I do not recall a single immediate post-operative death, although in the medium term death was often inevitable.

The experience for nurses in training was varied and challenging. Added to general ward duties, the fortunate ones spent substantial time in the operating theatre, where procedures, unusual to a general hospital, were seen. In the plaster room we were taught skills in the construction of plaster beds and turning cases for patients suffering from spinal tuberculosis - in which the patients were immobilised for a period of two years or more. The majority of limbs were also immobilised by means of plaster of Paris, a window cut out for the drainage of suppurating wounds.

The training regime for nurses was strictly rooted in the Nightingale tradition. The hours were long - call at 6 a.m., in the wards 8 a.m. to 8 p.m., two hours off-duty during the day, and lectures to be taken in off-duty time. Days off-duty were few - a half-day or full day off each alternate week, and two weeks holiday each year. The salaries started at £20 per annum in the first year, increasing by increments of £10 per annum. There were no deductions for meals or residence as these were 'all found.' Preliminary examinations for State Registration and for orthopaedic nursing were taken during the second of the two year course.

Discipline was absolute, to a level now regarded as absurd. Entry to any room, on or off duty, was in order of seniority, as was seating at meals. No conversation could be initiated with those of even slightly greater seniority. Despite such restrictions, which were largely regarded as an inevitable component of hospital life, the Royal Sea Bathing Hospital was a happy place. Strong leadership came in the shape of the Matron, Miss Rachel Kempson, and the Medical Superintendent, Basil Armstrong - formidable, charming and handsome and something of a legend in his day.

Efforts were made to protect nurses from contracting tuberculosis, mainly by means of an ample diet. BCG vaccination was not yet known. Nonetheless, several nursing colleagues did acquire the disease and two died in my time there.

We learned much and grew rapidly from girls to young women. We watched those with no hope show great courage and great comradeship. We viewed major orthopaedic surgery, and in the isolation block we nursed diphtheria, anterior poliomyelitis, and the dreaded surgical erysipelas.

Chapter 2
The Radcliffe Infirmary, Oxford
1937 - 1940

Thus equipped it was time to move to general training. Application was made to and accepted by the Middlesex Hospital in Mortimer Street, London. Fate, however, intervened. I had determined to marry a young officer leaving within days for active service in the then mandated territory of Palestine, a wifeless station. The Middlesex Hospital for its part had determined not to accept married nurses in training, nor to allow any remission in length of training time for certificates already held. Fortunately, the Radcliffe Infirmary, Oxford, which had a reciprocal arrangement with the Royal Sea Bathing Hospital, accepted me, and on 1st January, 1937, I arrived at the Radcliffe Infirmary Preliminary Training School in Headington.

Three months later his death on active service once more altered my hopes and plans for the future. Having arrived at the Radcliffe, it seemed sensible to complete general nurse training with a view to entering medical school at the age of 21. Description of life in Preliminary Training School would nowadays be greeted with total disbelief.

Elementary nursing procedures were interspersed with domestic tasks, the day closing with an inspection of laundered dusters carefully folded and displayed in an exact manner, draped over the sides of a small cardboard box. The harsh discipline was only fleetingly resented by the majority. In retrospect, it seems our self-regard was low. The suggestion was readily accepted that we were fortunate indeed to be allowed to train in Oxford, and that any flouting of regulations or rules would be followed by instant dismissal.

The Radcliffe Infirmary was a delightful and in some ways an eccentric repository for larger than life figures of medical and nursing staff. Discipline was strict, the regime rigid, and freedoms much restricted. Off-duty was frequently curtailed at the whim of a ward sister. Each day began with mandatory chapel attendance, and ended with prayers on the ward. In strict order of seniority we knelt on the polished ward floor, and woe betide any nurse on Marlborough or Rowney Wards who had the poor taste to permit a patient to call for urgent attention or to suffer a cardiac arrest in full flow of worship.

Two legendary ward sisters, who had served on the Western Front in the 1914 - 18 War, were the Misses Hitchcock, one now presiding over Men's Surgical, the other over a Men's Medical Ward. Each day their chauffeur drove them in their

81 VANDON COURT,
PETTY FRANCE,
LONDON SW1H 9HG
TEL. 071 2221414

PONSMAEN,
ST. FEOCK,
TRURO TR3 6QG.
TEL. 0872 862275

December 15th 1991

Dear Chak,

This book is being sold in
Cornwall for the Cornwall Leagues of Friends.
If we had it on sale at meetings of the
Cornwall Clinical Society, priced at £5 do you
think anyone would wish to buy it ???
If so who do you think I should approach?
I think Cath will find the early part
interesting!

With love to you both from
Belinda and Terry.

Daimler to the hospital. Once 'on duty' they communicated only through their terrified junior nurses and in the third person. As Rowney Ward was directly above Marlborough Ward, much time, effort and anxiety was spent in running up and down the granite staircases carrying missives of doubtful civility.

These were the days of pre-eminence for ward sisters, and their authority was absolute within their domain. Eminent professors and clinicians would not enter wards in advance of the customary courtesies, and all matters other than clinical treatment of patients - and much of that - was subject to their control. House officers failed to recognise this at their peril, but many owed much to the wisdom and experience of these women.

It is worthy of note that despite some astonishing and truly deplorable techniques, including the sharpening of lumbar puncture needles on the granite staircase (the needles then duly sterilised) the incidence of infection and cross infection was very low, almost negligible. Naturally this was of great importance in days before the ready use of antibiotics. To allow a pressure sore to develop in even the most debilitated patient resulted in a visit to Matron's Office, a reprimand and a note on the file of the offender.

Basic nursing care was taught and practised, as was the earliest concept of intensive care. A special unit was developed, attached to a surgical ward (Cronshaw) known as the 'hot box'. It was wrongly believed at the time that patients suffering surgical shock and others requiring intensive care, required nursing at a high ambient temperature of about 75 degrees.

Emergency admissions were attracted from a wide range of industrial accidents, including extensive burns occurring not infrequently in Morris Cowley Pressed Steel works. These patients required highly specialised medical and nursing care.

Sexually-transmitted diseases were treated in conjunction with diseases of the skin in Briscoe Ward. From the standpoint of nurses in training, work in this ward was both a crude and unpleasing introduction to matters sexual. Specially sought after was work in the general operating theatres, where a strict and very able theatre sister meted out training which stood us in good stead in subsequent years. Here I was fortunate to add to the extended time I had spent in theatre at the Royal Sea Bathing Hospital. And it was here I discovered that I would find my future as a nurse in surgical wards and operating theatres, though it remained my ultimate aim and interest to enter medical school.

Dressing packs and instrument packs were unheard of. Theatre linens were packed in separate drums as were abdominal packs, gauze swabs, gowns, caps and gloves, extracted by forceps as and when required. A trolley was set up in advance of each procedure with the 'general set', the necessary 'extras' for the particular procedure, and any other required equipment. Needles were set out on needle holders together with suture material, the nurse 'taking the case' having to thread the needles required. As time has passed, the introduction of theatre packs, dressing packs, Theatre Sterile Supply Services and Central Sterile Supply Units and pre-threaded needles, much has changed.

Nevertheless, nurses serving under difficult circumstances during civil unrest abroad, or under fire, have remarked on the need to 'learn' their instruments, rather than being able to rely on merely opening the requisite pack.

A 'Centre of Excellence'

Several coincident events conspired to transform the Radcliffe Infirmary in the late 1930s from a busy provincial hospital with an associated pre-clinical medical school, to a national and international centre of innovation and excellence. An endowment by William Morris, later Lord Nuffield, enabled the Radcliffe to build a new ward and theatre block to house the academic departments of neuro-surgery, anaesthesia, and gynaecology. This gift accompanied the appointments, in 1937, of Professor Cairns, later Sir Hugh Cairns, to the Chair of Neuro-surgery, and Pro-

Professor MacIntosh, later Sir Robert MacIntosh, to the Chair of Anaesthetics, together with their supporting staff. The appointment of Professor Chassoir Moir as Professor of Obstetrics and Gynaecology rapidly followed. Between them, these three specialists drew many others of skill and distinction.

Professor Cairns brought with him from The London Hospital, a highly trained operating assistant - Mr. Alibone - one of the first to be so trained. I recall Mr. Alibone accompanying the Professor on his ward rounds, the conduct of which was distinctly idiosyncratic. The customary retinue was brought up at the rear with a House Officer carrying a bread basket in which all manner of instruments required by the Professor were to be kept at 'the ready'. The 'bread basket rounds' are remembered to this day.

House Officers to the Professor complained that they were given little responsibility and little hands-on experience. As neuro-surgery was in its infancy and much still experimental, Professor Cairns's reluctance to delegate to junior staff is readily understandable. Certainly he inspired many who worked with him with immense loyalty and enthusiasm.

Sir Robert MacIntosh, a New Zealander, had qualified at Guy's Hospital, becoming a Fellow of the Royal College of Surgeons before an interest in anaesthesia led to his appointment at Oxford to the first Professorship in Anaesthetics in this country. Soon the Department of Anaesthetics at the Radcliffe became a meeting place for British anaesthetists, and for others from all over the world. With him to Oxford, had come his technician, Mr. Salt, from whom those of us working in theatres learned a great deal. At his instigation the speciality of Anaesthetic Nurse was introduced within the hospital.

Aside from writing extensively for the medical press, and publishing several books on anaesthesia, Professor MacIntosh developed some important pieces of anaesthetic apparatus. One of these was the *Oxford Vaporizer*, a particularly successful machine for the administration of ether, widely distributed to the Services through the continued generosity of Lord Nuffield, and of great value in World War II. MacIntosh also organised the distribution of Iron Lungs, given by Nuffield in 1938, to hospitals throughout Britain and the Empire.

John Stallworthy, now Sir John, joined Professor Chassoir Moir as Registrar on January 1, 1938. His arrival is vivid in my mind due both to his remarkable car - complete with fern growing from the rear seat - and to his delightful friendship. Sir John has left to posterity* a full account of the

---

*   'Radcliffe Infirmary, Oxford, 1937-8', in the **British Medical Journal**, Vol. 294, 16 May 1987.

discussions leading to Lord Nuffield's generous gifts to the Radcliffe and his rebuilding of the Wingfield Morris Orthopaedic Hospital, and the appointment, upon which he insisted, of Mr. Girdlestone as Nuffield Professor of Orthopaedics.

A Centre for people

These years were overshadowed by the Munich crisis followed by a brief period of ill-founded euphoria and then by the looming presence of the Second World War. Despite, or possibly because of the heightened sense of impermanence of life, as Munich came and went, followed by the increasing certainty of war, life at the Radcliffe when off-duty was far from dull, gloomy or stratified between medical and nursing staff.

John Stallworthy briefly described in his account the arrival of the Canadian contingent of junior medical staff from Toronto General, their gaiety and informality characterised by an 'easy come, easy go' approach to relationships with nursing staff who quickly recognised this propensity. Other members of the Medical Common Room were equally colourful. Gus (Edmund) Wigram, a member of the 1936 Everest Expedition, was also distinguished by reason of his marriage, hitherto unheard of in House Officers, to Kit, a nurse at St. Thomas' Hospital, London, herself a lively personality. Both Gus and Kit became close friends to many at the Radcliffe, and all of these were deeply distressed by Gus's later death, climbing in Snowdonia on his demobilisation leave.

Social life was transformed at the hospital by the appointment of Miss Margaret Bonthron as Matron upon the retirement of Miss Muriel Sparke. Miss Bonthron epitomised all that was best in the nursing profession between the wars, combining dignity with charm, and insisting upon the highest professional standards with explicit trust in each of her nurses - unless and until that trust was seen to be misplaced. To those who from time to time found themselves in great difficulty she was a compassionate and wise friend. Under her guidance a yearly Summer Ball was instituted in the Nurses' Home. So many other social functions were initiated that I recall being reminded as Secretary of the Social Committee that the Radcliffe was a hospital and not a social centre. It was saddening for us all when Miss Bonthron's fiance, who had been the Hospital Chaplain before joining the Army, was killed at Arnhem.

From those days, there are many others whose work, charm and individuality leap readily to mind: the unfailing courtesy of Mr. Abernethy, Honorary Gynaecologist, the calm demeanour of Dr. 'Crisis' Cooke, Honorary Physician, the humour and skill of Freddie Durbin, Resident Surgical Officer and later Consultant Orthopaedic Surgeon in Exeter, and the idiosyncratic determination of Professor MacIntosh to keep his weekly date in Paris for his dancing lessons. A lasting impression was left by Sam Corry, an Honorary Surgeon, Dr. Alice Carlton, Dermatologist, Dr. F. G. Hobson, Honorary Physician, and the father and son paediatricians, Drs. 'Pappy' and Ernest Mallam, successive coaches to the Oxford University eight.

The ghost of Lizzie Waddelove

Legends regarding supernatural manifestations persist in hospitals throughout the world. Certainly it is not surprising that a highly charged emotional atmosphere should prevail in buildings, the walls of which have contained the heights and depths of human experience. So it was that here at the Radcliffe walked Lizzie Waddelove. The Ear, Nose and Throat ward at the Radcliffe in the late 1930s, was housed in an up-graded part of the hospital formed of two wings, one for men, the other for women, with the operating theatre en suite between the two. I was on night duty in my last year of nurse training, and had never heard of Lizzie. Nonetheless, after many instances of hearing the approach of Night Sister, rising to meet her then finding no one there, over a number of weeks, I mentioned this phenomena to others who had worked in the hospital much longer than I. They told me about Lizzie Waddelove. The reason for her haunting was obscure but said to relate to the death of a child. The footsteps definitely resembled those of a woman - light and walking rapidly - but they never reached my desk.

A geographical footnote
Visitors to the Radcliffe Infirmary today would not recognise 'their' old hospital. The fountain remains, as does the Chapel, but the main entrance and the main corridor down which we raced with suitable decorum for hurried meals, is now altered so that entrance to wards leading off the corridor are concealed. There has been a widespread change of use of departments and operating theatres following the transfer of the majority of acute services to the John Radcliffe at Headington.

Chapter 3
Clinical Advances

The development of *prontosil* in 1938, followed by the *sulphanilimide* drugs M & B 693 and M & B 760, revolutionised the care of patients suffering from conditions previously regarded as likely to be fatal. *Puerperal sepsis* responded to these drugs as did *septicaemia,* and the later *sulphanilimide* drugs such as *sulphasuxidine* were used as 'cover' in intestinal surgery. Controversy and rivalry persists to the present time regarding the discovery and development of *penicillin* as between Oxford and St. Mary's Hospital, Paddington. In the latter, the very window sill in the Clarence Wing upon which Professor Fleming noted the remarkable properties of *Pencillium notatum* in September, 1928, is preserved and shown to visitors with immense pride.

Penicillin is the name given in 1929 by Fleming to an antibacterial substance produced by a species of mould *(Penicillium Notatum)*, which contaminated a culture plate which was planted with *staphylococci.* Fleming noticed that around the mould colony the *staphylococcal* colonies were undergoing lysis, thus he grew the mould in pure culture and studied the properties of the antibacterial substance-*penicillin*. Since that time, *penicillin* was used in the laboratory for differential culture, though early attempts to extract the active principle failed. It was not until 1939 that Chain, Florey and their co-workers at Oxford, succeeded in concentrating the *penicillin* sufficiently to reveal its remarkable chemotherapeutic properties. Many other moulds had been tested, and aside from *P. notatum* other members of the *Chrysogenum* group had been shown to produce *penicillin*, though not to the equal quality of *P. notatum*. Thus it is that from this mould all *penicillin* is produced.

In 1943 an article recording a series of 187 cases of sepsis treated with *penicillin* appeared in *The Lancet* following a remarkable case at St. Mary's Hospital, Paddington. The patient suffered from *meningococcal meningitis*. Having failed to respond to injections of *penicillin* at the recommended dose, he responded and recovered following the administration of *penicillin* injected intrathecally.

The impact of the availability of this powerful remedy in the treatment of serious and frequently fatal conditions cannot be over emphasised. Morbidity and mortality resulting from the following conditions was revolutionised: *pneumococci; streptococci; staphylococci;* the gas-gangrene group of organisms; *B. anthracis; C. diphtheria;*

actinomyes; spirochaeta pallida; spirillae generally; gonococci; meningococci.
Sir Douglas Black[1] recorded his own presence in the Nuffield Department of Medicine, Oxford, when the first therapeutic injections of *penicillin* were being given by Charles Fletcher. At that time, Sir Douglas was working on *haematemesis* and on plasma treatment of burns shock. The work of Professor Florey in developing *penicillin* at Oxford in 1941-2 is well documented in Gwyn Macfarlane's biography of the scientist.[2] An interesting sidelight to the work of Professor Florey appeared in an obituary notice regarding Professor R.J.V. Pulvertaft who died on 30 March, 1990.

"During the Second World War Pulvertaft was Pathologist to the 64th General Hospital in Alexandria until his seniority and military experience led to his appointment as Assistant Director of Pathology, MEF, with promotion to Lt. Col. commanding the Central Laboratory housed in the 15th General Scottish Hospital in Cairo.

Ever alert to new advances Pulvertaft interested himself in Sir Howard Florey's work on penicillin. He obtained from Florey a culture of his Pencillium and produced vast quantities of the mould floating on the surface of countless gallons of broth in pails, crocks and tanks all over the laboratory floor. The filtrate was applied to infected wounds of battle-casualties by some of the hospital's surgeons, who found it very effective by the standards of the day.

1   **Recollections and Reflections**, (1987) Cambridge University Press.
2   **Howard Florey, The Making of a Great Scientist**, (1979) Oxford University Press.

But this venture was frowned upon by Florey and his team, who did not want their work on the extraction of pure penicillin for systemic use to become confused with the local application of a crude brew. Three pundits flew out from England to investigate, but Pulvertaft defended his procedure so ably that all ended happily. (St. Thomas' Hospital Gazette (Spring, 1990)

It is important to recognise the amazing impact of drug therapy in the entire spectrum of disease in the nineteen thirties and forties. *Broncho-pneumonia,* 'the old man's friend', no longer brought death to those whose span of life was complete, children no longer died of quite common complaints, and child birth was seldom followed by fatal sepsis. It is salutary to remember the great advance and enormous relief gained through the use of the Salk vaccine and the later widespread preventative programmes for protection from poliomyelitis. Other problems resulted from increased longevity and lower mortality and morbidity, and these are mentioned later in this book.

Techniques covering intravenous therapy were improved during these years as were those of blood transfusion, cross-matching and the near elimination of adverse reaction following incompatibility. Blood transfusion was a relatively rare event and blood banks were unheard of. Donors were commonly a family member brought to the hospital for this purpose and placed in the adjacent bed. Citrated blood would be stirred with a glass rod as it was introduced through a venous cannula into the patient's vein, having been withdrawn from the donor through a needle with a butterfly phlange. In due course these elementary procedures were superseded by the glass vacolitre, the antecedent to the present donor envelope provided by the Blood Transfusion Service via the blood banks. Today's use of blood in relatively routine surgery would have been regarded as profligate in the extreme. For comparative purposes, the interested reader may wish to consult *Price's Textbook of the Practice of Medicine* [3] which provides a vivid description of procedures in use at the time, illustrating the then elementary state of the art. The restoration of body fluids following injury and shock was less fully understood pending great strides made during the Second World War.

3   By various authors, (1946) Oxford Medical Publications.

Chapter 4
The War Years, 1939-45

The certainty of war encouraged many of us to marry rather earlier than would otherwise have been the case, and my husband-to-be, then House Officer to Ronald Macbeth in the Ear, Nose and Throat (ENT) Department, left the Radcliffe with me in July, 1939.

By now I had achieved State Registration although my certificate was withheld for a while pending the necessary minimum age for registration. I had achieved four years of valuable experience in two markedly different institutions, mostly in surgical wards and operating theatres, and had survived the rigours of training under the discipline of those days.

The Armed Forces would not accept married nurses, therefore in August, 1939, I joined the Civil Nursing Reserve. On Sunday, 27th August, my husband received his call-up papers as a member of the RAF Volunteer Reserve Medical Branch. Together we travelled to London where he reported as instructed, only to be told that, as it was the weekend, he should return home and await further orders. War was declared the following Sunday, 3rd September, and again he departed, this time to serve in the RAF throughout the war.

The memory of foreboding broadcasts throughout the 2nd and 3rd September, 1939, will never be erased from the memories of those who listened. The inevitability of war had long since been accepted, but as always, hope died hard.

Upon hearing the fateful and now famous words of Prime Minister Neville Chamberlain, I set off from Wheathampstead to London in a small, open Austin 7 in order to take my husband's sister-in-law and her small son to safety. The outward journey was uneventful, the return journey interrupted twice by air raid sirens and a precipitous and totally unnecessary refuge in nearby ditches.

In the first few weeks of war, my duties with the Civil Nursing Reserve were terrifying. For the first time I found myself working in an unknown district, without friends, without colleagues and senior staff with whom to consult, and without knowledge of my husband's whereabouts from one day to the next. Equally without previous experience outside the safe confines of a hospital, the work I was called on to do was alien as well.

In the main, I gave cursory medical examinations to child evacuees, treated their minor ailments, and awaited the alarming prospect of the arrival of bus loads of expectant mothers, due or overdue, and many of these with abnormal presentations of their babies. A partially-completed roadhouse was commandeered for these purposes. The mothers arrived at intervals, and were examined before being billeted and delivered. Equipment was rudimentary in the extreme, trestle tables serving as examination couches, grey army regulation blankets as linen, and sterilisation accomplished by means of boiling instruments in fish kettles. All credit to the District Nurse that despite such adverse circumstances and my lack of midwifery experience, there were no obstetric disasters, no still-births or neonatal deaths attributable to my lack of skill during those first weeks.

Such good fortune seemed unlikely to continue. It was with great relief and alacrity that I accepted the invitation to return to the professional safety of the Radcliffe Infirmary and the Gynaecology Department with its attached operating theatres. Promotion was rapid, albeit by default since the Departmental Sister had been called up for service as a member of Queen Alexandra's Nursing Service.

Work at the Radcliffe during the first year of the war, known now as the 'phoney war' continued much as before though certain units experienced changes of use. The Churchill Hospital was opened for head injuries, many members of staff left for service with the armed forces, and the character of Oxford as a university town underwent marked change.

Perhaps the most astonishing event, well documented elsewhere,[1] was the transfer from Germany by air of Unity Mitford to the care of Professor Cairns, following a self-inflicted gunshot
wound to her head. Some fifty years later, Professor Fraenkel of the Department of Surgery, Flin-
ders University, South Australia, began to research the life and work of Hugh Cairns. In the
process he interviewed those of us who were present that evening, with particular reference to the
removal or otherwise of the bullet from Miss
Mitford's brain.

Strict confidentiality surrounded the flight from
Germany as arranged by Adolf Hitler, and the
subsequent admission to the Radcliffe. I remembered well the event, but could not recall a 'ping'
as metal dropped into the receiver. Following
further enquiries by Peter Morris, Professor of
Surgery at Oxford, it transpired that following
Miss Mitford's death her brain was preserved in
the medical museum. A fire later destroyed the
specimen, but it seems the bullet had not been
removed.

When seven months pregnant and no longer able
to wear a uniform, I joined my husband at the
RAF Officers Hospital, Torquay. The Palace

1   Price-Jones, David (1976) **Unity Mitford, A Quest,** Weidenfeld &
     Nicholson, and Guinness, Jonathan and Catherine (1984) **The**
     House of Mitford, Hutchinson.

Hotel had been converted to serve this purpose. Suddenly the reality of war was with me. Walking our small dog on Babbacombe Downs, I came under machine gun fire by a 'hit and run' raider. He flew low out of a cloud, and used up his unspent ammunition by spraying the ground indiscriminately, school children and I being the only targets. We lay in nearby ditches and all escaped injury. Sadly, such good fortune did not last. Shortly after, the Officer's Hospital was bombed with resulting casualties.

Before that our elder son was born, in the course of an air raid and without any medical attendance. We put him to sleep in an open wardrobe drawer, the two doors open to protect him from shrapnel. The day that he was born, invasion was thought to be imminent. Service personnel were to be moved inland, civilians to remain where they were. Service revolvers were issued to medical staff, hitherto unarmed, in order to protect their patients. Although this was the first real threat of invasion to this country since the Napoleonic Wars, it was received with true British phelgm. Beaches were heavily mined - many mines remaining until some time after the end of the war.[2]

---

2   An interesting account of the work of that hospital at the time is found in Chapter 7 of **From Where I Sit**, by Dan Maskell (1980) Collins.

My husband was posted to RAF Uxbridge in the autumn of 1940. Together with our baby son I joined him as the blitz and Battle of Britain were reaching a crescendo. I was able again to nurse and worked in various capacities throughout the war, notwithstanding the birth at two yearly intervals of two baby daughters.

Our home in Hillingdon became unsafe as the entire structure tilted forward at a 10 degree angle. The front door would not open, nor the back door shut, though surprisingly the house stands upright today. We moved to Gerrards Cross as the flying bombs and rockets battered southern England, sometimes reaching us when overshooting their targets. During this time I was fortunate to continue working in the relative safety of Civil Defence Control.

Much is written of the blitz and the Battle of Britain, the historic speeches of Winston Churchill as Britain stood alone following the fall of France and the Low Countries. Less is written about the utter dreariness of war on the home front, the fear engendered by the flying bombs, and the effects on morale of constant bombardment by the new weapon, the 'pilotless plane.' The sight of the latter in the sky is unforgettable with its tail of flame, flying in all weathers, undeterred by anything, and then the moments as the engine cut and silence preceded the explosion. Mercifully, these and Hitler's so-called 'ultimate' weapons - the rockets of Peenemunde - reached only the South of England and Greater London, though some overshot and fell as far afield as Oxford.

As time passes, much of the day-to-day activity and emotional impact of the war years is forgotten. I kept no diary but recall the acute pleasures in surviving each air raid or attack. Children, put to bed each night in siren suits ready for immediate evacuation, grew and flourished. Gardens bloomed. Though strict, rationing was adequate and fair. Nursing practice changed little.

A Defence Regulation precluded those who were trained nurses from working in any other capacity than nursing, but in the event I cannot recall such a wish on the part of a single colleague. As the war concluded, the survivors gave thought to future careers.

My husband was now totally committed to a future in ENT surgery, having spent some time towards the end of his RAF service updating his skills at St. Thomas's Hospital, London. As demobilisation drew near, he heard of an opening in Cornwall as assistant to Michael Sheridan, then recovering from prolonged ill health. To Truro we travelled on an exploratory mission, a journey never to be forgotten. Since Britain was still at war, the blackout remained in force.

At Plymouth we drew up the blinds of the night train and beheld the most desolate sight - a city razed to the ground. It seemed that no habitable building remained standing. Familiar as we were with the destruction and devastation wrought in London, we had no idea of the affect of saturation bombing on this small, high density city.

Chapter 5
After the War

The Beveridge Report published in 1946 had paved the way for sweeping changes in the social structure and social philosophy of the United Kingdom. That landmark prepared the way for the introduction of the National Health Service Act of 1946. Thinking people were fired with the vision of people free from financial anxiety, secure from 'cradle to grave' and health care free at the point of delivery. But, to achieve that vision, work was ahead.

We arrived in Truro on a bleak raw morning. The city was shrouded in heavy mist and appeared most uninviting to any other than a devotee of Cornwall. Such a one was my husband, committed since his childhood. For me, a move to Cornwall would result yet again in the frustration of my long held determination to study medicine. To pursue that desire I had been attending the (then) Regent Street Polytechnic to brush up on First MB and prepare for Second MB.

Little did I foresee, as rebelliously I travelled from Paddington to Truro on that and subsequent visits, how devoted I too would become to my adopted County, and how indebted I am to so many people from every facet of Cornish life. Even more unforeseen is the later commitment and debt - some thirty five years on - to the district surrounding Paddington Station and to St. Mary's, Paddington, and its associated hospitals.

In the months and years immediately following the end of World War II, daily life in a Cornish village was far from easy. During the war, despite the blitz and flying bombs in London, we were never without domestic gas for cooking, never without water, and seldom without electricity. Shops were near, as was a nursery school for the children. Daily help with the house and baby sitting was always at hand. In Cornwall none of these amenities existed. Day to day living was a substantial challenge therefore, and especially in the severe winter of 1946-47.

Back to Work

In the summer of 1946, my husband announced, "I have a job for you. They need a trained nurse to run Out-patients and Casualty at the hospital. I have arranged an interview with Matron for you!"

I hadn't worked in a hospital since leaving the Radcliffe, and my multifarious nursing experiences during the war had not fitted me for either of the posts. Nevertheless, holding the Matron in considerable awe, I duly attended for interview. Thus began one of the happiest, most satisfying jobs I was to hold - but not in Out-patients and Casualty. Instead I went to work in women's surgery, and particularly in gynaecology.

The hospitals of Cornwall in 1946 were staffed in the main by medical staff who, in addition to their hospital work, were also engaged in general practice in the locality. The Royal Cornwall Infirmary provided a full range of general services other than obstetrics and radiotherapy. The Redruth Miners' and District Hospital - always commanding great respect and loyalty from those living nearby - provided the full range of services including these. West Cornwall Hospital, Penzance, was essentially a sub-district general hospital. Falmouth and District Hospital provided general medicine, general surgery, gynaecology and a local accident unit. Tehidy Hospital treated patients suffering from pulmonary tuberculosis, of great prevalence at that time, in pavilion-type wards. Treatment there involved artificial pneumothorax and thoracoplasty with Mr. Griffiths, Mr. Belsey and Mr. Barratt all visiting from Bristol and London.

The East Cornwall Hospital at Bodmin, St. Austell and District Hospital, Fowey and District, Newquay, and Edward Hain Hospital, St. Ives, all provided a level of service which in later years was to be regarded as inappropriate and to some degree unsafe, due to having no resident medical staff. In essence these hospitals were cottage hospitals, greatly valued by the public and general practitioners alike.

An historical account of the outbreak of polio-myelitis in Cornwall may be of interest to some readers. In Appendix 1, a partial reprint is given of a report by Dr. E.R. Hargreaves who was then Deputy Medical Officer of Health for Cornwall County Council. In addition to spending much time caring for patients in the isolation unit at St. Clement's Hospital at Truro, where polio patients were treated, Dr. Hargreaves, known to his friends as Peter, was tireless in his efforts to comfort and reassure those families affected by this illness and to minimise a sense of near panic in the population at large.

My own work was to be with John Hood whose main field was gynaecology but who was also a GP practising in Truro. On re-joining, initially as a part-time staff nurse, I found little in nursing had changed. Prolonged bed rest following surgery was still routine. Early mobilisation of patients after their operations was not yet in vogue. Women's surgical, as it was then known, was run with great efficiency by Sister May Bennett, who had trained at the Royal Northern Hospital. Dressing techniques and nursing procedures were identical to those taught in my own training even though the advent of *penicillin* and the *sulphanili-mides* had revolutionised many aspects of treatment, and the outcome of disease. My work was unusual, and this was due to a severe shortage if not total absence of junior medical staff.

My responsibility was to 'clerk' patients admitted for gynaecological surgery, take blood if required, and prepare patients for surgery. Two days each week I would assist Mr. Hood with his operating lists in theatre - in the absence of a House Officer. The lists included the entire range of gynaecological surgical treatments including elective and emergency ceasarian section. Despite his size and his huge hands, Mr. Hood was an adept and gentle surgeon, calm and undeterred in the face of what he might find on opening the abdomen. I never heard him raise his voice in theatre, with the result that all who worked with and for him found it pleasurable. In addition to his general practice and work in the hospital, John Hood was an enthusiastic rider to hounds and a very colourful member of Cornish society, resplendent on the dance floor in hunting pink.

Like his colleague William Rentoul, an orthopaedic surgeon who had been decorated with the Military Cross, John Hood had served on the Western Front in the 1914-18 war. Undoubtedly, this experience was reflected in their willingness to tackle some surgical procedures which might well have daunted their peers. In addition to the experienced and efficient theatre sister, the mainstay of the general theatre was the porter, Mr. Lawrence, a mine of information and a mentor to junior nurses experiencing this type of nursing for the first time.

By 1950, the increased number of junior medical staff was again depleted with the outbreak of the Korean war where one of their number was killed. Here in Britain, petrol rationing and soap rationing came to an end, and other commodities became more readily available. That same year difficulties arose in recruiting a night sister capable of 'taking' theatre in addition to general duties. I took the job, initially for six months, but this stretched to a substantially longer period.

In 1951, I was again 'over-large for uniform' and left the hospital to prepare for the birth of our second son. Thus ended a seventeen year nursing career working directly with patients. It had been a privilege to help to care for them, and from them I took many lessons in how to live and how to die. From the many superb medical and nursing staff I also learned much.

The introduction of the NHS in 1948 had passed almost without comment in the hospital. The principal change was that former honorary members of the medical staff became salaried members of the Consultant Medical Staff on a full or part-time basis. Eleven sessions of three hours duration represented a full-time working contract for a consultant.

The medical contracts were held by the South Western Regional Hospital Board. All general hospitals west of Liskeard were administered by the West Cornwall Hospital Management Committee. It is noteworthy to mention that the numbers of consultant medical staff in Cornwall have risen dramatically - from 17 in 1948, to more than 80 in 1989.

Chapter 6
Related to Health, 1952 -1967

The irrationality of much of human behaviour had long concerned and interested me. The opportunity to learn more presented itself when the University of London introduced a Diploma in Social Studies, entry to which at ordinary degree level was by means of London Matriculation which I had obtained many years before. Though abated by earlier qualifications the study programme extended over a two year period, twelve months of which was spent in Child Care Services (then the Children's Department of County Councils), Child Guidance Departments and with the Probation Service.

The academic discipline and the chance to gain practical experience in aspects of life hitherto unknown to me, presented an exciting challenge. I followed this with an Honours Degree in Sociology, students of which have been much maligned and regarded as 'crazy lefties.' The academic course comprised papers in economics and at final level social administration, psychology, social history, criminology, anthropology and statistical methodology. After completion of the degree work in 1955, a relevant post with Cornwall County Council became available. My dual remit was to quite disparate fields of interest. Firstly I was required to conduct a survey within the County of the incidence of disability, having defined the various categories of disability and degree of impairment. Secondly I was to undertake a study of the services provided by Cornwall County Council in support of so-called 'problem families', and to make recommendations, to initiate, to organise and to manage an amended service geared specifically to the needs of these families.

The report was produced in 1959, and this, together with recommendations, was accepted in its entirety by the County Council. As a result a fresh concept of support and care for families in difficulty was introduced. Referral to this service, based in the Social Welfare Department answerable to the County Medical Officer of Health, was through Health Visitors or other professional staff, including the Probation Service and the Housing Departments of the Local Authorities.

In effect, this new service was a safety net. It aimed at the prevention of homelessness, by helping to avoid evictions following arrears or non-payment of rent and other unmanageable debts. It aimed to assist families, parents and children alike, by giving help to rectify poor hygiene habits and to promote healthy diets. Many families were housed in Nissen huts, formerly occupied by troops during the war and located in isolated and windswept sites. These were now surplus to requirement but out of the public gaze and away from all amenities including schools and shops. These were the 'ghettos' and carried that stigma.

The homes and gardens on housing estates were decimated, a plague of broken windows, tumbled walls and fences, cracked surfaces of every description. In some instances the external appearance mirrored internal and appalling standards of sanitation beggaring description on these pages. These required the help of the Public Cleansing Department before our staff could attempt to support and help the family.

To recruit the staff - to be known as Family Welfare Workers - a novel approach was used. The sole criteria was a robust and mature personality. The applicant could be of any or no professional background, and of no particular age group. The influence of the Younghusband Report on *Social Workers in Local Authority Health and Welfare Services, 1959,* should be noted. Recommendations included a recognition of the need for three grades of workers and for those working with clients with straightforward or obvious needs including a brief but well-planned in-service training.

The result was near miraculous due to several factors. Wholehearted support was obtained of the Housing Officers in the County, a rent guarantee scheme was introduced, and heroic efforts were made by the Family Welfare Workers. Evictions and thus homelessness was markedly reduced - almost to vanishing point - and children of families hitherto regarded as 'impossible to integrate' in normal society, became indistinguishable from their peers at school.

The sensitive approach of the Headmaster of one school was indicative of a new attitude: without drawing attention to the plight of some of his needier pupils, he made arrangements for them to wash and change into school clothes upon arrival so that no longer would they be shunned by their fellows. Certain aspects of the scheme could reasonably be described as social engineering.

The results, however, were immensely encouraging and cost effective. Eviction was prevented, loss of rent to Housing Authorities was avoided, costs were not incurred by the County Council through default under the Rent Guarantee Scheme, and not least, some interruption occurred in the general cycle of deprivation for these families. In contradistinction to the present time it is noteworthy that few families were headed by a single parent, the majority having a permanent relationship within marriage.

Many other changes in the social fabric have occurred during the decades following 1959, but the single overriding factor which emerges is the significant increase in single parent families and a concommitant rise in awareness of aspects of deprivation and sexual abuse, of which less was then known or recognised. During the years 1960-1966, the scheme grew, from an initial service offered to 24 families in 1960 to 123 families with 460 children under 16 years of age in 1966. Over that time only one eviction occurred, one boy was brought before a juvenile court, and one mother abandoned her children to be taken into care by the Children's Department.

Lest too rosy a picture emerge, it should be admitted that the adult clients appeared with depressing regularity before the Magistrates Court - usually for relatively minor offences - and one family in particular continues to appear as the generations pass by, so that grandchildren are now to be found in the Court previously graced by grandfather. So much for interruption to the cycle of deprivation.

Cornwall's scheme antedated the publication of the *Seebohm Report* which from the early 1970s made changes inevitable. The concept of the generically-trained social worker, who would be able to tackle all 'problem' areas was introduced, in contradistinction to the specialisations that had been previously promoted upon entrance to social work.

Special mention must be made of the work of Dorothy Watkins in Cornwall, where she served as County Children's Officer from 1948 to 1972. The County secured in her the services of a woman many years ahead of her time with high intelligence, great energy, enthusiasm and sensitivity. She had the ability to recruit and retain staff who were equally highly motivated. Her professional partnership with two leading members of the Probation Service in the County, Joan Channel and Neville Elcoat, ensured a level of care and guidance for the children and young people of Cornwall that provides a worthy example to those working today in similar fields.

In 1965, I left the employ of Cornwall County Council, having learned much about public life and the world of the 'submerged tenth'. To my immediate boss of those days, Frank Mountford, the County Welfare Officer, I owe the value of his oft spoken edict, "in public life when speaking or writing of an incident or an individual, always think of how this might appear in a tabloid newspaper". Wise words indeed, to which I would return many times in memory.

In the meantime I had been appointed to the (then) West Cornwall Hospital Management Committee and the (then) South Western Regional Hospital Board. In addition I had accepted substantial responsibilities as a Marriage Guidance Counsellor. The first two of these provide more 'snapshots' in this album.

Chapter 7
Health Services in Cornwall
1962-1977

My introduction to the new world of hospital management, with all its exciting new developments, came as the Health Service in Cornwall embarked upon a programme of building and rebuilding. The laying of the foundation stone of a new hospital to be provided at Treliske, Truro, in May, 1962, was presided over by Mr. Enoch Powell, then Minister of Health. This was a culmination of tremendous efforts and determination over a number of years on the part of the late Mr. William Rentoul, a Consultant Orthopaedic Surgeon, and Dr. Charles Andrews, Consultant Physician. They followed up the report published by the Ministry of Health in 1945, entitled *The Hospital Services in the South Western Area* which resulted in the formation of a Planning Committee in 1951. Mr. Rentoul and his colleagues had succeeded in persuading the Ministry of Health and the Regional Hospital Board of the need for additional hospital facilities in Cornwall, and the necessity for bringing these facilities into line with modern medicine.

At its first meeting the Committee recommended that a new hospital should be built on a site one mile west of Truro. A twelve and a half acre site was acquired, which in turn was increased by a further eighteen and a half acres in 1963, to permit the ultimate expansion of the projected hospital to approximately 700 beds.

Prior to the opening of Treliske, general medical, surgical and children's services had been especially fragmented, spread as they were between the Royal Cornwall Infirmary, Truro, the Redruth Miners' and District Hospital, and the West Cornwall Hospital, Penzance. Maternity services were provided at Redruth Miners' and District Hospital, and the Bolitho Hospital, Penzance. The needs of patients in the east of the county were provided for by the Plymouth Hospital Management Committee. Some acute and a large amount of sub-acute work was undertaken at eight general practitioner hospitals spread through the county, with the long term care of elderly patients in so called 'chronic sick' units at Perranporth, Budock, Poltair and Meneage. There were also hospital beds in Local Authority institutions.

In effect my first few years as a member of the Hospital Management Committee were an apprenticeship under the guidance of the then Chairman, Mrs. Joan Hain, and several other very wise and experienced 'elder statesmen'. From them I learned a great deal. These were the days of sub-committees and involvement of members in the day-to-day, detailed management of the affairs of the Health Service to an extent unrecognisable and unacceptable in later years.

The Group Secretary, David Preston, who had been Clerk to the Governors of the Westminster Hospital, was of the 'old school' of hospital managers, seeing himself as the servant of his Committee and of the Medical Staff. Other more superficial traditions were upheld such as the wearing of hats by women members of the Committee at all meetings. This habit continued until I became Chairman in 1967.

South Western Regional Hospital Board, 1965 - 1974

My appointment in 1965, as a member of the South Western Regional Hospital Board provided the chance to widen knowledge and experience in hospital services from Bristol westwards to the tip of Cornwall. During the years 1965-1974, the Chairman and 28 members of the Board operated through seven Sub-Committees which involved members in much travel throughout the area. Initially the Board was chaired by Colonel Arthur Guy. a most delightful person of great charisma who became a very dear friend. His courage in the face of death from cancer of the larynx was an inspiration to us all. He was followed as Chairman by John English, later knighted, who came to us from an entirely different background, namely the Electrical Trades Union. Sir John possessed similar qualities of leadership and courage in the face of his own serious then terminal illness in 1973.

Throughout the period the Secretary to the South Western Regional Board was Harold White, a consummate practitioner in the art of 'wheeling and dealing' in public life. He had an outstanding ability to achieve his objectives whilst the live characters on his chess board usually remained completely unaware of his strategy in the game. Harold was ably assisted by a strong team of medical administrators whose influence pre-1974 re-organisation (of the Health Service) was substantial and widespread. Several of these became close personal friends.

James Westwater, followed by Iain Sutherland, the two Senior Administrative Regional Medical Officers, Bill Davies and the late Rex Cheverton, two senior members of their staff, were all well known and well respected throughout the Region. The financial management and control of the affairs of the Board were ably directed by the Treasurer, Frank Rushton, and later by Trevor Rippington. If there was direct interference in regional matters by Central Government officials, this was substantially less evident than in subsequent years. Nevertheless, stringent control was exercised over capital and revenue expenditure of the 31 constituent Hospital Management Committees.

The general hospital services, the psychiatric hospital services and the mentally handicapped services were administered independently, each group under a Hospital Management Committee. The integration of the latter two specialties, mental handicap and psychiatry, developed gradually as the opportunity presented itself. Simultaneously, the Board under John English's chairmanship, attached great importance to the need to improve standards of care in hospitals for the mentally ill and mentally handicapped. A working party was set up under the chairmanship of a recently retired Physician Superintendent, with the wide remit to study existing services and to make recommendations for improvements. Initially such a study was thought of as 'threatening' by the hospitals concerned, but subsequently found to be of great assistance in ensuring a well-informed debate at Board level.

In looking over the Year Books for the period, the quality of members of the Regional Hospital Board and the constituent Hospital Management Committees stands out. The majority held both academic and professional qualifications and were men and women with wide experience. Party political affiliations appeared to play no part in the appointment of members to Authorities.

During these years it was usual for a number of chairmen of Hospital Management Committees to hold simultaneous appointments as members of the Regional Hospital Board. These appointments enhanced rather than diminished the ability of the Regional Board to allocate capital developments even-handedly across the Region, making use of the cumulative wisdom and experience of the local members.

The re-organisation of the NHS in 1974, with its preclusion of joint membership of both authorities, has seemed to many to have been unfortunate. That which had been based on the concept of partnership between Hospital Management Committees and Regional Hospital Boards - notwithstanding occasional tensions and difficulties - risked in 1974 a change toward an adversarial stance as between Regional, Area and District Authorities. With Regions, Areas, and in some places Districts as well, and chairmen, members and officers having to establish and understand their new roles, the practice of continued joint membership might well have avoided counter-productive tendencies.

Chapter 8
Change and Chairmanship in Cornwall

1967-1971 The West Cornwall Hospital Management Committee
1971-1974 Cornwall and Isles of Scilly Hospital Management Committee
1974-1977 Cornwall and Isles of Scilly Area Health Authority

Upon arrival in the Chairman's Office at St. Clements Hospital, Truro, I was assured by the gentle and courteous Group Secretary, that a Chairman could 'do anything'. With total naivety I accepted this amazing concept. It was a period of rapid developments in medical science, and subtle but marked changes in social structures and inter-professional relationships. There were also gradual but determined moves in defining the respective roles of Members and Officers of Health Authorities.

The affairs of the Committee were in some disarray. An unacceptable level of overspend threatened, and financial management had been poor despite the best endeavours of the previous Chairman. The health of the Group Secretary, David Preston, was giving cause for anxiety, and his condition was such that he could only work part-time. In 1969 it became necessary for him to retire from his post altogether, and in April John Goldsworthy from St. Mary's Hospital, Paddington, London, was appointed in his stead.

John brought with him a youthful freshness and enthusiasm which was unusually infectious. Coupled with his ability to command the devotion of his staff and the friendship of medical and other professional staff, his coming bode well for Cornwall. None could have foreseen the enormous pressures and tensions - emanating from integrations and re-organisations - with which he would have to deal, and which certainly would have daunted a lesser man. In the face of all the problems his courage and loyalty remained unshaken, and I as his Chairman owed and continue to owe him a debt which cannot be paid.

It was rapidly apparent that the Treasurer's Department needed strengthening to rectify a near disastrous situation. In Gerry Roberts, appointed as Group Treasurer, Cornwall gained one whose ability to persuade, cajole and influence people was second to none. He was, in truth, a Welsh Wizard, upon whom I came to rely entirely in matters financial. His ability ensured that at the end of each financial year's closure of books, there would be a miniscule balance, but never an overspend!

Despite financial problems these were years of rapid development in the Cornish Health Service.

The building of the Hospital at Treliske attracted young and ambitious medical staff determined to provide a first class service to the people of Cornwall, whilst reluctantly acknowledging that certain conditions could not be treated locally. Facilities for some specialist procedures simply could not be provided, and would have to be referred elsewhere.

Treliske Phase I initially offered 180 beds for general medicine and general surgery, together with supporting departments and staff residential accommodation. The first patients were admitted in May, 1966. Phase II provided 80 maternity beds, 20 special care baby units and an ante-natal clinic. Future developments promised to include departments for accident and emergency, outpatients, and paediatrics. At that time no mention was made of the need for gynaecology or the care of the elderly on the Treliske site. At May, 1966, the total cost of capital development was £2,912,000.

The Royal Cornwall Hospital, Treliske, was opened officially on 12th July 1968 by HRH Princess Alexandra, the Honourable Mrs. Angus Ogilvy. The opening was preceded by a prayer to Her Majesty the Queen, through the Privy Council, to allow for the use of the prefix 'Royal' in the hospital's title. In all matters pertaining to the Palace, the Lord Lieutenant, Sir John Carew Pole, and the Clerk to the Lieutenancy gave unstintingly of their help and counsel.

The Opening Ceremony was on a perfect summer's day and greatly enjoyed by all who worked to ensure its success. The events were tinged with sadness too, in remembrance of those missing. Tim Rutter, who had anticipated working as a general surgeon at Treliske, and who had performed the first operation in the theatres of the hospital, died shortly thereafter of a sudden, massive heart attack. Willie Rentoul, one of the main 'architects' of the project also did not live to see the embodiment of his hope for medicine and surgery in Cornwall.

Inevitably the euphoria engendered by the prestigious new building was punctured. The new facilities threw into high relief the inadequacies of the old as embodied in the Royal Cornwall Hospital, City, formerly known as the Royal Cornwall Infirmary. On the one hand those working at 'City' were the 'poor relations'. On the other, there were unrealised, perhaps unrealistic, hopes and aspirations on the part of those working at Treliske. In the event, it was the latter which gave rise to major anxieties and much unrest.

No sooner were the wards open and inhabited, than deficiencies in ward design became obvious, making difficult the observation by nursing staff of acutely ill or unconscious patients. There was a lack of monitoring equipment and other essential pre-requisites of modern acute medicine. An intensive care unit was demanded, followed by coronary care and a renal dialysis machine for use in acute renal failure. (In those years it was accepted that chronic renal failure would be treated at Plymouth.)

In answer to these expressed needs, a part of Ward Five (an acute medical ward) was converted to intensive care, another part to coronary care. The requisite cardiac monitors were provided through voluntary contributions due to determined efforts of Dr. Tony Thould and his colleagues. Likewise, the first renal dialysis machine was donated in 1969. Twenty years later it seems unthinkable that a new acute unit could be planned lacking these facilities now regarded as routine, but at that time, many now established techniques were in their infancy. Tony Thould was later instrumental in introducing a comprehensive rheumatology service to Cornwall. With his example, The Regional Hospital Board was persuaded to attach increased importance to this disabling condition so prevalent in the South West.

The Rheumatology Unit Trust at the Royal Cornwall Hospital (City) was provided by voluntary funds raised through the energy of many people inspired by Tony Thould. It was supported as in so many other efforts in the County by Lady Falmouth, Chairman of the League of Friends of the Truro Hospitals.

In November, 1967, an episode occurred which threw certain changes in public expectations of medical care into sharp focus. A road traffic accident resulted in the death of one of two sisters, the remaining sister receiving serious head injuries causing unconsciousness. Sadly, this girl was already severely mentally handicapped. Her subsequent treatment attracted a great deal of media attention and suspicion, the suggestion being that because of her mental handicap she would not receive all possible intervention and care. Television cameras appeared at the hospital entrance, medical staff were interviewed, and in order to reassure the public, the following statement was given to the press:

"The Medical Staff of the Hospital are delighted at the measure of recovery which has been achieved in this case and are proud that this hospital, with its Intensive Care Unit, can offer the necessary facilities for patients gravely injured and seriously ill throughout the County.

This girl was admitted to Treliske from the Accident Department at the City branch of the hospital at 6:30 p.m. on the 18th November, 1967, deeply unconsious and showing signs of severe brain damage. A tracheostomy was performed because of her comatose state in order to maintain her airway, and she was ventilated post-operatively for a few hours, after which she was breathing adquately under her own power. She continued gravely ill for six days with a very high temperature and frequent spasms. These were controlled by the normal method of drug therapy and cooling.

On the 25th November because of involuntary over-breathing and muscular spasms, which were causing exhaustion, she was put on a breathing machine for a short time. Additional measures to control her respiration and involuntary movements were required. She was therefore given a paralysing drug which necessitates use of the breathing machine.

At no time during the patient's stay in the hospital was she totally dependent on the breathing machine except as a result of the paralysing drugs which were deliberately used to control her exhaustion and which could have been reversed at any time enabling her to breathe under her own power. Treatment throughout was determined solely by medical considerations.

The Medical Staff and the Hospital Management Committee would be pleased to meet representatives of the press to clarify any outstanding points which they may wish to raise."

(reprinted in various newspapers such as *The West Briton and Royal Cornwall Gazette,* and the *Western Morning News*)

The above experience was unprecedented in Cornish health service activity, and we learned a great deal from it, not least the difficulties for medical and nursing staff in reaching decisions under the gaze of television cameras.

Chapter 9
Visitors, Strife and Achievement

Visitors...

In 1967, Her Majesty The Queen, the Duke of Edinburgh and their teenage children Prince Charles and Princess Anne, on the latter's first official visits, honoured the hospital on St. Mary's, Isles of Scilly. It is significant to note the change in the level of security precautions taken between that visit in 1967, and a subsequent visit by the Prince of Wales in 1977 to the same hospital. On the earlier occasion, security was minimal despite the presence of the Sovereign and the heir to the throne. In 1977, conscious that the Isles of Scilly constitute the first landfall from the Republic of Ireland, every drawer was opened, the roof space inspected and every part of the hospital examined scrupulously by Special Branch and their sniffer dogs.

In September, 1969, the Minister for Health, Richard Crossman, visited Cornwall. A lunch with consultant medical staff at Treliske gave opportunity for a forceful but good humoured exchange of views. The consultants anxiously regarded the current state of the NHS, mentioned the pressure on acute beds, and were countered with alacrity by Crossman's concerns about their earnings from private practice. Except for the difference in political persuasion on the part of the Minister, the 'conversations' could well have served as a rehearsal for the 1989 exchange of views between Kenneth Clarke and the medical profession.

Thinking of Richard Crossman, several 'snapshots' come to mind. He impressed those he met on that visit as a man of high intelligence with a quick grasp of essentials - but also unpredictable. In the evening of Mr. Crossman's visit a dinner was given in his honour at County Hall. The Minister had been greatly impressed by Dr. Tom Wilson, a Consultant Geriatrician and demanded that I arrange that he be invited to dinner and seated near him. This seemed to cause great dismay in terms of protocol, however we prevailed. At lunch, he had caused a minor sensation when during a moment of total silence which tends to afflict these occasions, he turned to me and boomed "Tell me, Chairman, are you sexually sophisticated?" The assembled company awaited my reply breathlessly. In fact his query related to educational opportunities for his son and daughter in what he perceived as an increasingly permissive society.

In remembering Mr. Crossman, it should also be recalled that the Health Advisory Service was formed at his initiative, and his contribution was major to the improvement of hospital services for the mentally handicapped. The quality of service and the level of enlightenment about mental handicap was uneven at that time. I recall the shock I felt in visiting a hospital some distance from Cornwall, in the course of which I saw a severely handicapped and blind patient lying totally naked on a dunlopillo mattress in a single cell-like ward. On the same occasion, in the patients' dining room I observed a naked female patient in the midst of others having their supper. Always self-evident to me is the dehumanising effect of poor physical and social conditions on both patients and carers. Conditions obtaining in a number of hospitals for mentally ill and handicapped people were indeed deplorable, notwithstanding the heroic unsung efforts of many staff members.

These cases were brought to a Special Meeting of the Regional Hospital Board and supervisory and management changes were made to ensure such conditions would not continue. In this - and other similar efforts - we were greatly helped by Crossman's determined programme of refurbishment and replacement of outmoded and totally unsuitable accommodation by Crossman Units, single storey, purpose-built buildings.

HRH The Prince of Wales included Treliske in the itinerary of a 1970 visit to the Duchy. He indicated a wish to visit departments rather than wards, and a programme was arranged which included a visit to the operating theatres. A Consultant Surgeon, the late Roy Adlington, renowned as an extrovert capable of dealing with any unexpected situation, approached a patient who enthusiastically agreed to allow his gall bladder to be removed under the royal gaze. At a given signal the incision had been made, and as the Prince reached the observation corridor, the abdominal towels were in place and contents exposed. Everything proceeded with exemplary precision. On noting some Princely pallor, I found it expedient to limit the time spent admiring Mr. Adlington's skill, and we moved rapidly to our next destination. The Midwives formed a Guard of Honour as the Prince left the hospital, and book was made as to which of the many attractive girls he would single out for a word as he passed. Bets were won that day as he chose the two anticipated to attract his attention.

A visit by Sir Keith Joseph in 1973 to the Royal Cornwall Hospital (City) and Budock Hospital, Falmouth, was a great encouragement at the time. Whilst on tour in Cornwall, Mr. Edward Heath visited Barncoose Hospital, Camborne, during a period of industrial unrest. A small but vociferous demonstration greeted him, masterminded - it was alleged - by known dissidents from outside the County.

A time of strife...

Valuable as the above visits were, and grateful as we all were to those who concerned themselves enough to visit the hospitals in Cornwall, discontent amongst medical staff at all levels and unrest among nursing and ancillary staff was increasing daily and threatening to overwhelm the service. Ancillary pay was extremely low, some with gross pay of £19 per week, though the Unions alleged even lower levels. The Regional Hospital Board Chairman, himself a Trade Unionist, charged us to do all we could to improve the pay of these workers within the regulations. We tried, but little could be done.

A demonstration and march was organised in November, 1972, with some 600 staff approaching the City Hospital where I was to meet them. This was years before the infamous 'winter of discontent' and we were relatively inexperienced in dealing with such manifestations of unrest. On the day of the march I had been advised to wear a bright colour, to position myself where I could be seen, and to stand my ground. Consequently I wore a red raincoat and stood on the steps of the hospital. As the shouting crowd approached it appeared as if an ugly scene might develop. Just at that moment when confrontation seemed inevitable, a window from the operating theatre complex above me opened, and a member of the medical staff emptied a receiver full of urine over my head.

The demonstrators were so outraged by this unseemly behaviour that from that moment onwards and throughout my term of office as Chairman in Cornwall, industrial relations were conducted with utmost courtesy. This does not mean that there was ever a lack of robust determination on both sides.

The early 1970s were a time of almost constant unrest. Discontent erupted from time to time in what became known as 'industrial action', and for the first time action was taken by consultant medical staff. Reasons for the latter's action were complex and included a sense of being undervalued and held in low esteem by the government. Salaries and wages had come to a standstill, the starting salary of a full-time member of the consultant medical staff in February, 1975, was £5,433. This stanstill resulted in the erosion of differential between senior medical and senior nursing and other staff. The following extract from a *Western Morning News* press report serves to illustrate.

A Report to Cornwall Area Health Authority has shown that Consultants' pay is lagging compared with salaries earned by other professions in the hospital service. The report by Chairman Mrs. Belinda Banham, follows the consultants' work-to-contract - now in its sixth week.

Their action has swollen hospital waiting lists and increased waiting time for some appointments from weeks to months. In her report, Mrs. Banham details current salary scales which demonstrate that other professions have overtaken medicine, in some instances to a marked degree.

For instance, minimum pay for a full-time consultant, at £5433 is £726 more than the salary paid to a principal medical laboratory technician, but £972 less than the earnings of an area nursing officer - and considerably less than the £7128 minimum salary paid to the area administrator.

The scales show also that the principal technician earns more than twice as much as a senior radiographer and £1000 more than a senior registrar on the medical staff.

Mrs. Banham says it is appreciated that there are intrinsic difficulties in formulating a contract which would be totally acceptable to all hospital medical staff. Nevertheless it is strongly felt that there must be recognition in respect of the many duties - on call, emergencies, night work, etc. which are at present undertaken without financial reward.

It would seem from the statement made by the Secretary of State on February 17, that she is giving due consideration to this matter. It is likely to prove impossible to price items of service if it were desirable so to do. However I am informed that at the present rates of remuneration of consultant (general) surgeons, for the performance of a major operation such as partial gastrectomy (removal of stomach) a surgeon is paid less than £5 and for all emergency work at night and weekends, no remuneration is received.

At the Authority's meeting at Truro last week, Mrs. Banham commented on the industrial troubles that were likely to beset the National Health Service for some time to come. She emphasised that staff and officers could do a great deal to mitigate the effect of action and make sure that personal relationships were not impaired.

The publication of the *Salmon Report (The Senior Nursing Staff Structure: Brian Salmon, Chairman, 1966)* had led to fundamental changes in the structure of the nursing services. The new nursing management hierarchy was not readily understood or accepted by the medical staff. In addition the continual, grinding shortfall in resources against rising demands fuelled dissatisfaction throughout the country. In Cornwall, the standard of care for patients admitted to Treliske had reached an unacceptably low level, and junior medical staff and senior nursing staff joined their voices in a chorus of rebellion on behalf of the patients. Under prevailing poor circumstances, it became clear that unless substantial changes were made, the standard of nurse training would be irrecoverably damaged.

Protest meetings were held which I attended. From these I established routine meetings with junior medical staff at both branches of the hospital, City and Treliske. The object was to enlist their support in managing the crises which arose. I invited a senior physician to act as referee on a daily basis should disagreement arise over 'placements' for individual patients. Consultant medical staff were supportive to these steps and the junior medical staff entirely cooperative in joint endeavours to bring order out of chaos. These meetings also highlighted dissatisfactions such as lack of recreational and dining facilities, and some of these deficiencies could be rectified.

Despite best endeavours, the situation deteriorated. Patients were being moved from ward to ward or discharged early and without warning. No continuity of care was provided, even basic nursing care became impossible in the shortage of acute beds, and the absence of good patient care was approaching the scandalous. This could not continue, and my own personal determination to demand assistance for both patients and staff was re-inforced by an incident which occurred in the foyer of Treliske.

A young man, lying on a trolley, was clearly dying of respiratory failure in full view of passersby. His mother stood helpless beside him. I was told that no bed anywhere in the hospital was available. Due to a design fault, there were no admission rooms and no separate entrance for ambulance cases. All traffic used the one entrance. The young man died. Despite discovering that he had congenital heart disease and was unable therefore to withstand a virulent chest infection, the situation was nightmarish and haunting. The sight of this dying patient in a hallway, his distressed mother alongside, and the desperate concern of the medical and nursing staff goaded me to extreme measure.

Meetings with the Secretary of State were held at six monthly intervals on the 16th floor of Alexander Fleming House. One such meeting occurred in December, 1972, immediately after the young man's death. On that occasion I asked to see someone of sufficient authority - someone whose decisions would effect change to a desperate situation. If this proved impossible I would sit all day in the corridor until someone was available. After some time, the presence in the corridor of a Chairman being clearly an embarrassment, I was transferred to the Minister's personal office - at that time belonging to Dr. David Owen - where I sat precariously on the edge of a chair. When it became clear that I wasn't going to leave Alexander Fleming House until I told the story of Treliske and the plight of the patients I was introduced to Professor Macdonald, head of the newly established Operational Research Department of the DHSS.

On my return to Cornwall, I sought belated approval of my actions from the Regional Hospital Board. A team from the DHSS under the direction of Bert Holdaway and Dr. Ross Tristem visited Cornwall with Professor Macdonald to initiate a study of alternative and optimum use of existing resources, both capital and revenue. The DHSS imposed the requirement that recommendation arising from the study should not lead to additional financial provision. Despite initial disappointment at hearing this, full support and involvement was obtained in the hospitals to begin the study in April, 1973. The results of this study are summarised in a paper prepared for a North Atlantic Treaty Organisation conference in 1976 with the theme *Systems Science in Health Care.* Appendix 2 contains a letter from me to the Minister of State for Health and Social Security (1975), concerning the values of the study to the Cornish health services, and a partial reprint of our paper.

Dr. Tristem and I presented our work in Paris based on the operational research carried out in Cornwall. The Canadian contingent had insisted that each paper was to be in both French and English. As I was allegedly bi-lingual it fell to me to present ours, though the greater part of the work and the authorship is attributable to Ross. Later he continued his interest in health and social care by assisting John Banham to set up the Audit Commission for Local Authorities in England and Wales. Now, in 1990, he is their Director of Studies as the Commission has been assigned responsibilities within the NHS in addition to their original remit to Local Authorities in England and Wales.

...and some achievements

Three individuals of outstanding dedication, vision and determination should not be forgotten in relation to ensuring that Cornwall would be one of the first countries to follow the example of Dr. (now Dame) Cicely Saunders, O.M., in providing hospice care for terminally ill people in the final stages of their illness. The late Countess of Mount Edgcumbe, the late Gordon Bellingham and the late Mrs. Enid Dalton-White assisted by a small steering group, many valiant fund raisers, several voluntary organisations and generous individuals, overcame local anxieties about the revenue consequences of such a scheme.

Dame Cicely had visited Cornwall and addressed a meeting in the Foster Hall, St. Lawrence's Hospital, Bodmin. Following this she kindly invited me to spend a brief time at St. Christopher's Hospice in Dulwich, so that I might observe their practice of patient care, and understand the concepts about which she spoke. As a result of the visit, I became totally committed to the project for Cornwall.

Mount Edgcumbe Hospice opened to its first patients in 1980. The appointment of Macmillan nurses followed closely upon that opening, the appointments funded initially by a generous benefactor. Since that time the work of Mount Edgcumbe Hospice and the Macmillan Nursing Service has grown and flourished throughout the county, bringing succour and comfort to countless patients and their families.

...and good works

The unbounded enthusiasm of the many members of the Leagues of Friends throughout the County was responsible for raising finance in support of countless projects large and small, and for much personal service to patients. The High Dependency Unit at the West Cornwall Hospital, Penzance, many Day Rooms and extensions such as those at Newquay and Fowey hospitals are just a few of the projects funded during these years. At St. Lawrence's Hospital, Bodmin, and its associated hospitals, the Leagues of Friends provided not only material support but most invaluable personal service and friendship to patients and staff alike. Cornwall was and remains in the vanguard in terms of fundraising activities for valuable projects and Trusts such as the Leukaemia Trust, the CAT-Scan Appeal, and latterly the First Air Ambulance. Services for the disabled based at Tehidy and St. Michael's Hospital, Hayle, under the leadership of Dr. Chris Evans have excelled. There seems no bottom to the pockets of the generous in the county of Cornwall. It is refreshing and invigorating to learn in 1991 that the first Community League of Friends in the country will join with the many other local hospital leagues in the newly named Cornwall and Isles of Scilly Leagues of Hospital and Community Friends which benefits the county so much.

...and feats of courage

During my ten years of Chairmanship in Cornwall, I was aware of many examples of outstanding personal service on the part of staff in all disciplines to the care and treatment of patients. Two especially vivid memories, which called for strong emotional courage, stand out in my mind.

The first is of a storm of such ferocity that it removed the entire roof of the service block at Treliske, creating both a hazard in terms of flying particles and in leaving essential services open to the elements. Tom Sixt, the Area Engineer, insisted upon climbing up to secure the necessary tarpaulins himself during the gale.

His feats were at considerable personal risk, as ropes could not be fixed anywhere to anchor him. He had served in the Merchant Navy throughout the Second World War, and regarded this current exploit with customary 'Geordie' phlegm. The subsequent award to him of an MBE gave us all immense pleasure.

My second memory is of the remarkable rescue effected by Cornish ambulancemen, and is best described in the following report made to the Health Authorities.

Cliff Rescue at Cligga Head, Perranporth

In the course of their duties, the Authority's ambulance staff find themselves involved in difficult and dangerous situations. A recent incident is, however, thought to call for special mention to the Area Health Authority.

On 23rd June, 1977, at 12.27 p.m. Ambulancemen W. Cocking-Jose and I. Inwood were called urgently to an incident at Cligga Mine, Perranporth. On arrival they were met by a policeman who said that a German potholer had fallen down a shaft. Coastguards and police officers were in attendance and after reconnoitring the situation the coastguards prepared to send men down for a rescue. Ambulanceman Inwood volunteered to accompany them.

The entrance to the mine was about 200 feet down the cliff where there was a ledge from which operations could be carried out; it consisted of a hole about 3 feet in diameter leading to the main tunnel, the full distance being some 300 feet with a 90 degree bend after 100 feet. At the end was a cavern known as Cathedral Cavern beyond which a shaft approximately 50 feet deep at the bottom of which the injured man was lying. Mr. Inwood was lowered and on examination found that the patient had wounds to the head and possible fractured ribs. The patient who was approximately 15 stone in weight was manoeuvred on to the stretcher and hauled up the shaft. This operation had to be carried out perpendicularly owing to the lack of space and cause the patient to vomit. Mr. Inwood immediately had him lowered again so that his airway could be cleared. Following this he was raised successfully and brought from the tunnel to the ledge outside, where he was picked up by helicopter and taken to hospital. For a considerable time the coastguard and Mr. Inwood had to sit in darkness at the bottom of the shaft and were eventually brought up with great difficulty.

Mr. Inwood has commented that the cooperation between coastguard, police and ambulance staff was excellent. Previously he had gone down a cliff only during an exercise for refresher training and he considered this later experience to have been of value to him. He was commended by HM Coastguard for his expertise in attending the injuries and his assistance throughout the rescue. During the operation which lasted 4 1/2 hours the ambulance management at the surface was carried out by Mr. Cocking-Jose who was responsible for relaying messages."

These incidents serve as a stark reminder, if such were needed, of the many and varied demands made upon the public services and the Health Service in particular.

Angry 500 get hospital tea
–and sympathy

1972.

CORNWALL'S lo
500-strong thro
and were offered tea
Committee's chairm

Hospital report spotlights salary margins

HOW CONSULTANTS HAVE MISSED OUT

Health Authority has shown that consultants' pay is
ies earned by other professions in the hospital service.
s, Belinda Banham, follows the consultants' work-to-
ek.

hospital waiting lists and increased waiting time for
s to months. In her report, Mrs. Banham details current
ite .... dicine, in
leg

Nurses' action begins to bite

THE work-to-rule by about
800 nurses in general and
psychiatric hospitals throughout Cornwall began to bite
yesterday, when it was
announced that probably at
least one ward at St. Lawrence's Hospital, Bodmin—the
county's largest—will have to
be closed.

But with the announcement,
from Cornwall Area Health
Authority chairman Mrs. Belinda
Banham, came an assurance that
no patients would be discharged.

She said : " We have four acute
admission units and will probably
move the patients from one into
the others. The action we take
will be without detriment to
patient care."

Mrs. Banham spoke soon after a
Bodmin meeting of the 22-strong
central co-ordinating committee of
the union involved, the Confedera-
tion of Health Service Employees,
whose work-to-rule decision was
taken on Monday.

NO PLANS TO SACK NURSES OR CLOSE HOSPITALS

CORNWALL'S Area Health Authority ha
no plans to close any of 'its' smaller ho
pitals or to create redundancies amon
nursing staff.

This assurance was given by Mrs. Belinc
Banham, chairman, at the authority's meetin
at Truro last week, when she commented o
a warning about possible effects of ove
spending voiced at a meeting of the region.
health authority a few days earlier.

Pointing out that reports of the Region
meeting had referred to overspending in Devo
and Cornwall "that might result in a need '
close small hospitals and create redundancy i
nursing staff," Mrs. Banham declared :

Chapter 10
The Elderly in Cornwall

Early Steps toward "Care in the community" and Hospital Services for the Elderly in Cornwall, 1960-1977

In the years following the Second World War acute medical care of elderly patients in Cornwall was based in general hospitals and local cottage hospitals. Additionally, there were some direct admissions of patients to long-stay hospitals in Redruth, Budock, Helston, Penzance, Perranporth and St. Austell. Lamellion Hospital, Liskeard and St. Mary's Hospital, Launceston were managed by Plymouth Hospital Management Committee.

Before the establishment of the NHS, the late Dr. Charles Andrews, a Consultant Physician to the Royal Cornwall Infirmary had conducted a survey of the public assistance institutions in the county as at 1946. His Report, presented to the County Council in 1947, led to the formation of a countywide geriatric service and the appointment of a specialist physician, Dr. Tom Wilson, as a Consultant Geriatrician in 1948, the first such appointment in England.

Taking this Cornish 'first' as an exemplar programme, Dr. Andrews visited Canada in May and June of 1953, speaking at meetings in Toronto,

Ottawa and Hamilton, about steps being taken to keep old people in their own homes, and the primary importance of diet in sustaining health in old age. At Montreal he took part in an 'institute' on geriatrics under the auspices of the city's Council of Social Agencies. The theme for the conference was the 'expanding hospital team', including not only the doctors, nurses and therapists, but the social workers, community nurses, neighbours, family and voluntary agencies.

In the mid-1960s, Dr. Andrews, together with other colleagues, persuaded the Royal College of Physicians to establish a committee with special responsibility in respect of medicine for the elderly. This was to become the Faculty of Geriatric Medicine of the Royal College. At the same time, Dr. Andrews, who had been a member of the South Western Regional Hospital Board since the inception of the NHS, exercised far-reaching influence over policies related to developing hospital services in general, and for the elderly in particular. One such development was of the first purpose-built psycho-geriatric assessment unit with associated day hospital in the United Kingdom. This was constructed on land adjacent to Barncoose Hospital, between Camborne and Redruth, and remains today an Acute Admission and Long-Stay Unit for the care of the elderly.

Such developments led to remarkable changes in attitudes toward the care of elderly patients generally, and more specifically toward the confused elderly. Though these are gradual and immeasurable changes of social attitude, optimism and professional appreciation of the importance of such home and hospital service have been acknowledged in numerous and public ways. The dread of being 'put away to Barncoose' or sent 'up Bodmin' has gradually faded and there is frequent recognition of both hospitals as providing a high standard of professional care, and without the stigma attached to public assistance institutions or lunatic asylums.

Succeeding years saw continuous and sustained improvements and initiatives in both facilities and policies related to services for the elderly and the confused elderly. Wards were upgraded, bed spaces improved and importance attached to protecting the privacy and dignity of individuals. The important contribution made to these improvements by enrolled nurses and nursing auxiliaries and of nursing assistants in those hospitals associated with St. Lawrence's, Bodmin, is especially worthy of mention, as is the leadership of senior nursing staff, notably Rhoda Weir at Barncoose and her colleague at St. Lawrence's, Alan Blythin.

Two wards for confused elderly patients were opened in June, 1973, with an associated day care unit at Penrice Hospital, St. Austell. The 'Sir John English' and 'Harold White' wards were officially opened by Harold White, Secretary of the South

Western Regional Hospital Board, and followed the earlier provision of a geriatric unit on the Penrice site. The building for the geriatric unit had been the first constructed in the United Kingdom using the Department of Health design employing the device of a compendium of component parts. Much was to be learned from that particular experimental design, not least that when cubicle curtains were drawn, ventilation was virtually non-existent. Patients and staff alike were subjected to unpleasant living conditions, and made changes and adaptations urgent and essential.

The Unit for the care of confused elderly patients was staffed and administered from the parent hospital at St. Lawrence's, Bodmin. This arrangement offered the welcome and well used opportunity for staff to exercise personal responsibility and initiative in the care of profoundly disturbed elderly patients within a more general hospital atmosphere.

The medical and nursing staff at St. Lawrence's were constantly campaigning for improved facilities for the elderly confused. In March, 1974, I opened the Norman Ward Day Care Unit in the Foster Building, and this development owed much to the initiative of Norman Ward, a Charge Nurse, who had conscientiously worked for higher standards of care for patients and for the maintenance of a good morale amongst staff in difficult times. Sadly, Norman died shortly after the Unit opened. In August of the same year, a Day Hospital for the mentally ill, and particularly the elderly mentally ill, was opened at Trevillis House, Liskeard, by Dr. David Owen, then Minister of State.

Purpose-built accommodation in the east of the County, as an alternative to acute admission at Barncoose, was opened in 1975 in the form of the 'Sir John English' and 'Hubert Dingle' units. Initially the beds in these units were used by the psychiatrists for confused and demented patients, but later were available to the elderly in general.

The ten years from 1967 to 1977 saw a gradual but nonetheless dramatic change in the entire concept of care for elderly patients in general and confused or demented elderly patients in particular. This specialty simply had not existed when I entered the nursing profession, and it had evolved virtually in isolation - through years of misunderstanding and neglect on the part of those intensely concerned with the acute hospital services. This was a development in the care of an increasing number of patients with which I felt particularly privileged to be associated. The medical and nursing staff in this field of work showed qualities of leadership and determination which served as an example, not only to other parts of the United Kingdom but to places far distant.

Chapter 11
Services for the Mentally Ill and Mentally Handicapped

Cornwall and Isles of Scilly Area Health Authority
St. Lawrence's & Associated Hospitals, 1971 - 1977

For many years hospitals for mentally handicapped adults and children in Cornwall were managed by the Royal Western Counties Hospital Management Committee (HMC) based at Starcross Hospital near Exeter. In keeping with the policy and philosophy of the South Western Regional Hospital Board to merge the management of psychiatric and mental handicap services with that of general services, the management of hospitals in Cornwall for mentally handicapped people was transferred in the first instance to St. Lawrence's HMC and then in 1971, together with St. Lawrence's and associated units to the newly formed Cornwall and Isles of Scilly HMC. My appointment in 1970 as a member of the St. Lawrence's HMC while serving as Chairman of the West Cornwall HMC, was followed in 1971 by being appointed to the Chairmanship of the newly formed and merged Cornwall and Isles of Scilly HMC.

In 1970 the St. Lawrence's HMC, under Hubert Dingle's chairmanship and the guidance of the Group Secretary, Stanley Smith, a start was made in removing the high perimeter wall surrounding the hospital and patients, hitherto hidden from public gaze. Thereafter those people who had been 'up Bodmin', as it was colloquially known, emerged and were to be seen walking in the grounds and later in the town. This was an early precursor to the current policy of care for those who are mentally ill or who have learning difficulties being provided in and by their own communities. But, this was just the beginning of a formidable task.

Re-furbishment of many wards was an urgent need; re-flooring was imperative in many instances to remove the stench of urine impregnation from many years use. Wards were of dormitory design, with little space between beds, and even less privacy. Sluices, bathrooms and lavatories were of nineteenth century design, totally inconducive to human dignity, and utterly discouraging to staff. Not only the physical surroundings needed re-building, so did morale. The staff had been subject to extensive inquiries into alleged cruelty to patients. All of a similar nature, these investigations became known as the 'Sans everything' inquiries and followed the exposures of certain appalling examples of maltreatment in hospitals up and down the country.

The St. Lawrence's Inquiry found some substance to the allegations made, and legal proceedings ensued. It therefore fell to management and the HMC to improve the physical surroundings thereby providing appropriate circumstances for proper standards of care. This was an onerous responsibility, demanding time and effort - in the first instance to win confidence and respect from the staff, and to allay their fears that a takeover was in store from the general and acute services management. Secondly it was necessary to persuade the Regional Hospital Board to allocate capital and revenue to up-grading wards, providing new buildings, and funding the necessary establishment of nursing staff and support services.

As Chairman of the newly formed HMC I had little or no experience in the management and administration of psychiatric and mental handicap services. The Group Secretary also had limited experience in this area of work. We found ourselves dependent in large measure upon the ex-Chairman of the former St. Lawrence's HMC, and the senior members of the professional staff of the hospital.

This was also a time of major change for the Medical Committees as the former concept of medical superintendency moved to new 'Cogwheel' concept of management arrangements. And it was therefore fortunate that when retirement of the Group Secretary of the former St.

Lawrence's Committee occurred, a senior member of his staff, Michael James, remained and was subsequently appointed as Administrator. A search for the post of Chief Nursing Officer to the new HMC was set in train, and John Green was appointed, having served with distinction on several national committees, including the Salmon Committee on Nursing. He had come from the post of Chief Nursing Officer at Moorhaven Hospital, near Plymouth, which was regarded at the time as one of the principal examples of good practice in psychiatric medicine and nursing.

Good fortune appeared in ample measure for the newly formed Cornwall and Isles of Scilly HMC. John Green was a Chief Nursing Officer in whom the nursing staff at St. Lawrence's and Associated Hospitals could have absolute confidence. Michael James had the wide experience, tact and wisdom of an Administrator, and was ably supported by Tony Sandry whose entire career had been committed to the Hospital. The medical staff, despite their own internal tensions, had confidence in them all.

As Chairman I was able to call on the advice and willing support of Hubert Dingle, and those of his colleagues transferred from the former St. Lawrence's Committee to the new HMC. With the constant help of the S.W. Regional Hospital Board, the Chairman Sir John English, and his officers, we faced many major problems with determination and enthusiasm.

An early problem was the need to improve the dress and personal hygiene situation for patients. The need for such basic items as tooth brushes and hair brushes was urgent, and steps were taken toward the introduction of a personalised clothing service. In the early 1970s this was considered an ambitious innovation - but the sight of these people lacking even the most elementary tools for their own care, and the concommitant lack of expectation on the part of staff who looked after them, determined me and the management to rectify this appalling institutionalism and deprivation. The positive support of the nursing staff, and the corresponding improvement in morale, gave us success in great measure. Special note should be made of the Professional Executive Committee, which included representatives of medical, nursing and administrative staff, and which to some degree took over the role and function of the former Physician Superintendent.

Few District General Hospitals in the early 1970s provided an admissions unit for acute psychiatry. The placement of such a unit in Ward 9 at the Royal Cornwall Hospital (City) along with an associated day hospital, was a vanguard action in this respect, and aroused some anxiety. Mainly controversial due to its geographical location in close proximity to wards for ENT patients and children, worries were assuaged only by a high ratio of staff to patients, time and absence of untoward incident. The Day Hospital opened within the main hospital grounds was yet another forward step towards integrating psychiatric services with general medical services.

Sir Keith Joseph, then Social Services Secretary, visiting Cornwall in October, 1973, commented as follows:

"I have been very impressed above all by the people I have met - bright eyes, enthusiastic, humane, dedicated people - doctors, nurses, social workers, occupational therapists....Cornwall has the same range of problems as the rest of the country on the social side, plus a bit more, because it has got more elderly than most places."

He had visited Budock Hospital that morning and seen the warm hearted care of mentally handicapped adults. He had also seen the old people's wards where he found, despite a good standard of care, a lack of diversionary activity or occupation. "But, this was known, and people were trying to do something about it," he commented.

"I went on to the City Hospital at Truro and saw the famous Ward 9, which is a pioneering job. Instead of waiting for the great new psychiatric wards that will one day be added to the new Treliske Hospital, this hospital has converted one of its own wards to provide acute psychiatry treatment. Here again I was filled with admiration by the enthusiasm and the team work."

'Marvellous' was the one word used to describe the new assessment centre for handicapped children. And, commenting on the age of the buildings at Budock, he said that "it was the combination of staff, purpose and team work which put them in the top rank."

Inevitably, there were risks taken amongst the many developments incorporated in order to remove barriers to freedom from earlier thoughts and strictures surrounding care for the mentally ill and handicapped. The risks however were backed up by strong nerve on the part of all staff, and a wealth of experience with the patients. Despite the presence in St. Lawrence's Hospital of patients from secure hospitals, all wards were kept unlocked, except in the event of seriously disturbed admissions.

In November, 1973, an incident occurred which was without precedent at the time. A middle-aged man suffering from paranoid jealousy had killed his wife by strangulation, and been committed on the order of the judge to hospital, under the Mental Health Act rather than to prison. Every hospital in the South and West of England was approached in order to comply with the direction of the Court, but to no avail. At St. Lawrence's, it was decided to call in the staff and seek their approval in advance of an agreement to admit the patient. In Foster Hall, all members of staff gathered -

medical, nursing, portering, domestic, engineering and ground maintenance.

The medical consultant, under whose care as responsible medical officer the patient would be admitted, explained the problems which might be encountered in providing appropriate care for this man. After assuring staff that there would be no compulsion to work with this particular patient, it was decided on a show of hands to agree to his admission. The staff were pleased that after fulfilling the undertaking made to the Court and the Department of Health to admit, observe, and assess the patient, he was safely transferred to a hospital nearer his home.

Services for mentally handicapped adults and children

As with the mentally ill prior to 1971, the services for the mentally handicapped (now known also as those with learning difficulties) had been managed by the Royal Western Counties HMC, and in-patient hospital provision was based at Starcross Hospital, Exeter. This had made the maintenance of family links for Cornish patients difficult, if not impossible, in many cases.

A record of developments and advances in caring for these patients cannot by itself tell the dramatic stories of how individuals were affected by changes made. One remarkable example is found in the story of Henry, aged 58, who had never been known to speak or express himself in any fashion. With the introduction of music therapy and art therapy, he began to paint, to use colour in imaginative ways, and also to play the guitar. These new interests evoked in him an evident desire to communicate, and in faltering but recognisable speech he told of his sister's farm and something of his early life.

This example both shamed and determined the onlookers and therapists and the reasons are obvious. Why had 'society' been so ignorant of the needs of people who admittedly had limited ability but could make some progress in self-realisation? We had to be determined to work for those services and facilities needed by Henry and others - to give them their chance.

A milestone in the treatment of handicapped children was achieved in 1972, under the auspices of the Cornwall Branch of the National Spastics Society and through the generosity of the people of Cornwall. A Counselling and Assessment Centre was opened for them in the grounds of the Royal Cornwall Hospital (City). The objective was to provide day-to-day support, on-going treatments and therapies, and any other appropriate care to children from the time of diagnosis until the age of admission to an education establishment. Initially the Centre was under Health Authority control and staffed by health personnel, but in due course the facility was transferred to the Local Authority Education Committee.

The architectural design was exciting and imaginative, and the Centre was constructed in a series of hexagons, which could be easily extended at a later date. The British Red Cross Society, as part of their centennial year celebrations, funded an adjoining hostel available to parents of the children attending the Centre for assessment. This was a forward move in helping to support parents coming to terms with their predicament.

The children attending the Counselling and Assessment Centre suffered from a variety of disabling conditions which included both physical and mental (learning) difficulties. For those children who exhibited learning handicaps (and frequently these were combined with physical handicaps as well), three in-patient hospital units were established. Two units were opened in 1972, at St. Blazey Gate, St. Austell, and at Loreto House, Bodmin. The latter was opened within 62 days to replace a private hospital closed as unsuitable. The change of use at Loreto House required the direct intervention and approval of His Holiness the Pope, as it was Catholic property. Subsequently I received a Christmas card from the Vatican. Then in 1976, Mrs. Peggy Jay opened Carn Brea House, Redruth.

It was with delight and encouragement that an excellent report was received by the Health

Authority and the staff concerned, following a later visit of the Committee of Enquiry into Mental Handicap Nursing and Care. The Chairman of that Committee of Enquiry was also Mrs. Peggy Jay. Subsequent events and changes of policy have led to further changes in use of these units, and to a greater emphasis on care for the handicapped in the community. During the years in question, however, these three hospital units embraced both a philosophy and a policy well in advance of their time.

These developments in care for the mentally ill and the mentally handicapped, owe their advancement to the efforts of many - the senior nursing staff, the medical staff, and not least the enlightened administrators. The re-organisation of the NHS in 1973-4 led to the establishment of the Cornwall and Isles of Scilly Area Health Authority. The substantial managerial changes resulted in the retirement from the service of the Administrator of St. Lawrence's and Associated Hospitals and later of the Mental Health Services, Michael James. As enabler and facilitator of much needed change, Michael's role cannot be exaggerated. The service owes him a great debt.

Chapter 12
To London to work

The years from 1977

After ten years as a Chairman in the Cornish health authorities, from hospital management committee (HMC) to area health authority (AHA) the time came to move on. I had been appointed Director of the Disabled Living Foundation, situated in Kensington, and this required that I live in London during the working week. The change was far from easy. The role change from Chairman of a large health authority, with its wide variety of responsibilities and interests, and the attendant social occasions, to that of employee away from friends and family was isolating and often lonely. To bridge this gap two previous activities came to my aid. I continued to serve as a Magistrate in Cornwall, and was also a member of the Industrial Tribunals in London (South). Aside from these bonuses, however, my sense of loss in 'leaving Cornwall' approached that of bereavement.

Fortunately, within weeks of arriving in London, I was invited to interview for membership in the Kensington, Chelsea and Westminster Family Practitioner Committee (FPC). The interview was conducted by Dr. John Dunwoody, then

Chairman of the local AHA and Tony Kember, then the Area Administrator. I had met Dr. Dunwoody previously in his earlier capacity as Member of Parliament and Parliamentary Private Secretary to the Minister of Health, Kenneth Robinson. I am grateful to them both - Dr. Dunwoody and Tony Kember - for giving me the opportunity to take my first step on the health services ladder in London.

For two years from 1977, I acted as a general member of the FPC, and learned something of the intricacies of the 'Redbook' (*Terms and Conditions of Service governing medical and other professional contractors*). During that time I was elected to chair both the Dental and Medical Service Committees, and then in 1979 was chosen by my colleagues to be the Chairman of the Kensington, Chelsea and Westminster FPC. Early in 1981 I was approached by Dame Betty Paterson, Chairman of North West Thames Regional Health Authority (RHA), and asked if I wished to be considered for a Chairmanship of one of the new Health Districts to be created by the then projected second re-organisation of the NHS.

The management arrangements created in 1973, as a result of working party recommendations (led in substantial measure by management consultants, McKinsey Inc.) were proving unsatisfactory, especially in multi-district areas. A management structure based on the idea of 'consensus management' by both District and Area teams of officers caused role confusion. Decision-making proved difficult, and there was frequently-voiced criticism. The proposal therefore was to abolish AHAs altogether, and in multi-District Areas to establish several small autonomous District Authorities answerable through RHAs to the Secretary of State. The difficulties experienced in these multi-District Areas had been much less evident in a single District Authority such as Cornwall.

To my great delight I was appointed to Paddington and North Kensington Health Authority as Chairman, and thus began one of the happiest periods of my professional life. Simultaneously continuing as Chairman of the FPC gave me invaluable insight and appreciation of the complexities and difficulties of general medical practice in the inner city. The help of an experienced administrator in Leon Screene, and the loyalty and friendship of professional and lay members of the FPC, opened the doors to my new endeavours. This convinced me - and I remain convinced - of the need for executive and non-executive managers in the NHS. All should learn, preferably at first hand, about the problems, opportunities and demands made upon general medical practice, and especially in metropolitan areas.

My experiences in inner London were a world apart from the conditions from which I had come in Cornwall. Twenty-nine percent of the 77 general practitioners (GPs) practicing in Paddington and North Kensington in 1985, worked single-handedly, compared with 12% in England and Wales as a whole. Thirty-nine percent of these doctors were over sixty years of age, a number over seventy, and several over eighty.

Initially, there had been a reluctance on the part of GPs to work from the Health Centres and gradually their reservations were overcome. Home visits presented enormous difficulties in some instances, and personal danger upon occasion. Lifts were vandalised in high-rise tower blocks, and mugging and other threatening behaviour not uncommon. Homelessness became increasingly recognised as a major problem; perceptions of it changed markedly, as it was realised that homeless people were not an homogenous group, but many individuals from different backgrounds and with varied social, economic, health and personality problems.

Young people arriving at Kings Cross Station, escaping what they believed to be intolerable home conditions or beckoned by what they expected to be a bright, high lifestyle, had little understanding of the hopelessness ahead if housing and employement were not already arranged. Prostitution and the drug trade might just as easily loom as the only means of livelihood. Multiple and various factors led to the presence in the city of older, homeless men and women with a wide range of health needs which were not being met by traditional medical services.

'Walk-in' Medical Centre, Great Chapel Street, Soho

The Department of Health sponsored and funded a pilot scheme in 1978, which immediately attracted clientele of both sexes and all ages to a "walk in" surgery in Soho. The medical care was administered by Dr. David El Kabir, a remarkable GP practising in Bayswater, who is also Fellow and Tutor in Medicine at St. Peter's Hall, Oxford. After assessing the results of the pilot scheme, the clinic was taken into the NHS with responsibility vested in the Kensington, Chelsea and Westminster FPC.

By 1983, Dr. El Kabir became overwhelmingly convinced of the needs of homeless people and determinedly committed to alleviating their suffering. He approached me as Chairman of the FPC and the DHA with a view to establishing some form of in-patient facility for those too ill to return to their cardboard boxes and shop doorways, but not sufficiently ill to warrant admission to hospital. He asked for premises declared surplus to Health Authority requirements to be made available to him - a large Victorian house in a run-down part of North Kensington. Concerns were necessarily expressed about what was thought to be the eccentricity of his proposal, and his seemingly unwarranted idealism. The plan was for medical students and junior medical staff from St. Mary's Hospital, Paddington, known to him at Oxford previously, to look after the sick men in a sickbay in the basement of the building, with accommodation above. The care of the patients would be provided free of charge by the doctors and students but payment for their accommodation, food and other essentials was to be met through their Social Security entitlement.

After prolonged negotiation as to premises, Wytham Hall Ltd. was established in 1984, and became a registered charitable trust supported by voluntary contributions and grants from other trusts. The medical staff, medical students and administrative staff became 'Members' of Wytham Hall, giving unstinting care to a succession of patients suffering from a wide spectrum of medical conditions both physical and psychiatric, and including in later years, those with AIDS. Notwithstanding their ongoing medical employment - as students and doctors in general practice - these medics have to date distinguished themselves academically as well as by their service. This fact has laid to rest any reservations I initially expressed to the Dean of the Medical School when the project was proposed.

As time passed, the need for a mobile surgery to service homeless people became apparent.

People sleeping out on the Embankment and in the Bullring underneath Waterloo Station required help. In 1987 a vehicle donated by the London-Edinburgh Trust was adapted and ingeniously equipped as a mobile surgery, and ambulance 'runs' were organised setting out at 8 p.m. on two evenings a week. That work required great sensitivity to gain the confidence of those who might come for advice and treatment; no addictive drugs were carried so the risk of violence was minimised.

It is unlikely that Wytham Hall could be replicated exactly elsewhere, as it has depended in great measure upon the leadership by example and precept of David El Kabir and those who work closely with him. Naturally it is hoped that succeeding generations of medical students and junior medical staff at St. Mary's and Oxford will wish to continue the practice of current 'Members' - finding each patient as 'a whole person' in need of care and treated as such rather than as a clinical problem to be solved.

Chapter 13:
Paddington and North Kensington

The ethnic background of the population served by the new Authority was diverse, and remains so. These are people from the old Commonwealth, the new Commonwealth and many European countries - as well as second and third generation 'minorities' born here. They present special health problems and some difficulties in health care delivery. Statistics from 1984-5 showed that 37.5% of the population in Paddington and North Kensington were born outside the United Kingdom, in comparison with 6.7% country-wide. (Source: *1981 Census*)

Reportedly, 56 different languages and dialects are in current use, and this alone makes the provision of health information in clear form a major problem. Cultural differences and religious beliefs require particular sensitivity on the part of all who treat and care for them.

On the *Jarman Index (Composite Index of Social Deprivation)* the area ranked as the most deprived District in the North West Thames Region, and the fourth most deprived in the country. In the index developed by the Department of the

Environment, it ranked as the second most deprived District in the country, Tower Hamlets alone being deemed even more so. Additional difficulties were created by the extreme mobility of the population. In certain parts 62% of those between the ages of 16-24 years, had moved in the year prior to the 1981 Census. Clearly we had problems.

The new Paddington and North Kensington Health District had, prior to re-organisation been a District within Kensington, Chelsea and Westminster AHA. A large measure of continuity of administration was fortunately secured by the initial appointments of three senior members of the 'old' Team, namely Terry Hunt as Administrator, Dr. William Kearns as District Medical Officer and Catherine McLoughlin as Director of Nursing Services. Stan Griffiths from Hillingdon joined later as District Treasurer, and Stan Holder, the much respected Director of Nurse Education, was a reassuring presence. As the new Chairman, simply 'imposed' upon them, I was necessarily apprehensive about the job ahead. Not least was I concerned about the wide variety of political perspectives amongst the Authority membership. But, though I quailed in prospect, I came into office on 1 April, 1982, and was welcomed and supported with great kindness.

Initially there were three people whose guidance was essential and most gratefully received. Joe

Bennett was the Vice Chairman of the Authority, a widely respected figure within the NHS, who had been secretary to the former NW Thames Regional Hospital Board, and to the National Staff Committee for England and Wales. He had been a member of the previous Kensington, Chelsea and Westminster AHA and the FPC, and he brought to the work of the new Authority an intimate knowledge of both problems and individuals. Terry Hunt as District Administrator was tireless in his determination to ensure the success of the new Authority. His commitment to the area and to St. Mary's Hospital was complete, and his wisdom and restraint in times of stress was beyond price. Finally, the late Pam Rooffe, my Secretary, whom I shared with Terry Hunt, was a mine of invaluable information. She had worked at St. Mary's from the age of sixteen, and through many years for Alan Powditch, the former Clerk to the Governors. Pam knew everyone and their idiosyncrasies and on countless occasions saved me from potential disaster.

I owe so great a debt to members of the staff both in academic and service departments in the hospitals, that it isn't possible to record every name - though some are mentioned through the text. International and national medical figures were numbered amongst the staff at St. Mary's. George Bonney was well-known for his work on the brachial plexus, Sir Roger Bannister as physician and athlete, Hugh Dudley as Professor of Surgery, Professor Sir Stanley Peart as Professor of Medicine, Sir George Pinker as the intrepid obstetrician - delivering amongst others of the European royal families, the Princes William and Harry. Alisdair Fraser, Nigel Harris, Geoffrey Glazer, Oscar Craig and Robert Elkeles became friends and colleagues. To all of these and many others I remain eternally grateful for the support and friendship generously afforded to me when I arrived as a stranger in their midst.

My Chairmanship of the DHA was concurrent with the Chairmanship of the Kensington, Chelsea and Westminster FPC until 1985, when Robert Davies was appointed to that position by the Secretary of State. I then remained as Chairman of the Health Authority until April, 1986. Throughout my tenure, I had the good fortune of support, counsel and advice from the tirelessly wise Max Lehmann. Amongst his many duties he had the unenviable task of taking the Minutes of the Authority throughout long hours of bitterly fought debates as we set about implementing controversial government policy.

The 'winter of discontent' had left a substantial legacy of poor industrial relations and a measure of real bitterness, despite the best endeavours of David High, a senior member of Terry Hunt's staff, and of John Geach, the District Personnel Officer. The Joint Staff Negotiating and sultative Committee was not working well, and there was little confidence and even less enthusiasm evidenced by either side. Implementation of government policy and the requirement to contract out various support services in addition to the need for strict measures to contain revenue expenditure within budget, served to increase the influence of activists within the staff committee. And a crescendo of complaints was reached during the miners' strike of 1984-5.

At open meetings of the Authority, I found the gratuitous insults hurled from the body of the audience hard to tolerate - and especially when they were aimed at members of the medical staff serving on the Authority. Also intolerable was the jostling and pushing that Members suffered approaching the Boardroom for their meetings. In those months of unrest I made several serious errors of judgment which could have resulted in disaster. Two such occasions spring most readily to mind.

In the first incident, some staff representatives demanded 'to see the Chairman' at about half past five one evening. Terry Hunt tried to dissuade me but I over-ruled his advice and a substantial number of staff together with an indeterminate number of activitists not in our employ poured into the Boardroom and steadfastly refused to leave throughout the evening. I then made a further error and allowed a table which had formed part of a hollow square to be removed as a result of which we lost control and the police were called. Twice I asked the protesting audience to leave the building and was met with refusal. At third request the police forcibly evacuated those remaining to the pavement in South Wharf Road. This was an appalling scene, mercifully not witnessed by other members of the Authority, which terminated some five hours after it began. My memory is not one of fear, but of shame and sadness that such an occurrence could take place within the Health Service as I had known it.

A second vivid memory related to the debate on the 'contracting out' of hospital support services. Public demand was such that the assembly hall of North Westminster Community School, north of the canal had to be employed for size. The debate concluded with a vote of 7 - 7 requiring a casting vote from me. It is generally accepted that a casting vote is used in favour of the status quo, but on this occasion it was imperative that the motion to proceed to invite tenders for support services was accepted by the Authority. Forgetting the live microphone I said, as though to myself, "well I am appointed by the Secretary of State and I owe loyalty to him", and my hand went up amidst furious turmoil. To their great credit, the Trades Union shop stewards in attendance stood between the platform and the body of the meeting and raised their hands to hold back the crowd, so no harm came of my unwise remark.

These were only two of the events which made a police presence - in a mini-bus ill concealed behind a wall adjacent to the Board Room - a requirement at every meeting of the Authority during these months. This was distressing and disturbing. I read genuine hatred in the eyes of some of the staff activists, and had never previously experienced such depths of animosity. In due time, as the miners strike and the print workers'dispute at Wapping drew to an end, the major leaders of disruption either left to pursue their interests elsewhere outside the district, or to further their professional careers in a less controversial manner. Well before my term as Chairman came to an end, a routine police patrol was no longer necessary.

Personally I learned much from these encounters, the principal lesson being the need to avoid any show of anger or distress. To fail to remain calm and in command of both emotions and events is simply to invite further disruption and to encourage a lack of respect for all authority.

Chapter 14:
Changes and Developments

Paddington and North Kensington Health District progressed from strength to strength during the years 1981-6, with the help and support of North West Thames Regional Health Authority, initially with Dame Betty Paterson as Chairman, succeeded by William Doughty (now Sir William), with David Kenny as Regional General Manager. The plans for capital development and rationalisation of acute services were conceived under the previous administration of Kensington, Chelsea and Westminster Area Health Authority (AHA), and owe much to the skill, foresight and enthusiasm of Terry Hunt, District Administrator of the North West District of the former AHA. These have continued steadily, culminating in reports produced in 1989 by the successor Authority, Parkside.

In 1981-2, it seemed that some question marks hung over the future of St. Mary's. This was evident notwithstanding the high reputation of the Medical School and the support of the Committee, chaired by Lord Flowers, on the future of medical education. Professor Peter Richards, the Dean of the Medical School and Evelyn de

Rothschild, the President of the School Council, were unsparing in their energies and enthusiasm to ensure a future for the School itself. Various options were explored and have eventually resulted in substantial investment by the Ludvig Institute for Cancer Research and the integration of St. Mary's Hospital Medical School with the Imperial College of Science and Technology. The new institution was inaugurated in 1988, and in that year the Medical School Council, of which I was a member, was delegated to the newly formed integrated Council.

In 1981-2 acute services were provided from three general hospitals - St. Mary's, Praed Street, St. Mary's, Harrow Road, and St. Charles' - with all associated administrative and treatment costs on three separate sites within one and a half square miles of each other. Gynaecology and opthalmology were accommodated at the Samaritan and Western Opthalmic Hospital in Marylebone Road. These services remain there, pending the full implementation of the acute services strategy which is to concentrate all acute services on the South Wharf Road site.

Prior to 1981, it was agreed to sell St. Mary's, Harrow Road, (initially, less the Woodfield Wing) together with almost the entire site. The sale would allow a substantial contribution toward the Queen Elizabeth, the Queen Mother Wing at South Wharf Road. From 1981 closure of Harrow

Road was scheduled for 1986, at which time the new Wing was commissioned and now accommodates general surgery, accident and emergency services, paediatrics, radiology and some parts of the medical school. St. Charles' Hospital has remained as an acute hospital providing a broad spectrum of services, although the Authority predicts necessary changes as the acute services strategy progresses.

Coming as I had from Cornwall, where services were necessarily available in one location at great distance from almost everywhere, I found it difficult to understand the fierce resistance of people in North Kensington in particular, to projected change of use for St. Charles' Hospital. The idea of centralising accident and emergency services and children's services was a cause of great anxiety. To try to understand the problems, I spent some time travelling by public transport, especially late at night, from the less salubrious parts of North Kensington to Praed Street - and, tried to imagine doing it with the additional burden of a toddler or two and a buggy. Quickly I was able to equate one mile across London at night to thirty miles by car in Cornwall and understood that though the difficulties were different in kind they were just as worrying to patients and their families.

Community Services and the Care of the Dying
In 1981, Chepstow Lodge - the first Community
Hospital in inner London - situated in Bayswater,
was a bright jewel in the crown of the former Area
Health Authority. Twenty-two beds were available to patients who were looked after by their
own General Practitioners. Not all local GPs par-
ticipated in this innovative scheme but those who
did were enthusiastic, and continued to provide
this care when Chepstow Lodge was sold and the
patients transferred to upgraded accommodation
on the Harrow Road site in 1985.

Adjacent to Chepstow Lodge, 42 beds ostensibly
for convalescence, rehabilitation and terminal
care, were provided at Hereford Lodge. The care
of the dying, though dedicated and caring, had not
progressed in line with the increased knowledge
and expertise of the modern hospice movement.
Initially through the personal generosity of a Cornish philanthropist, new 'King's Fund-developed
beds' were purchased for Hereford Lodge, which
delighted the nursing staff. The same Cornish
benefactor took steps to interest Cancer Relief
and the Macmillan Nursing Services in the care of
the dying in this area, and resulted in the appointment of a specialist medical consultant and Macmillan nurses for the unit.

The Health Authority came to an agreement
with Cancer Relief to share expenses for improved services. The Authority would provide

newly-upgraded accommodation on the Harrow Road site, the cost of patient care and support services, and the charity would provide a generous grant in respect of a medical salary and those of the Macmillan nurses.

In 1985 the Pembridge Unit of 22 beds was opened in the newly upgraded Woodfield Wing at Harrow Road, together with day care and community care services. The District was fortunate in its appointment of Dr. Anne Naysmith as the medical consultant in care of the dying and pain control, at a time when these specialities were in their infancy and few fully trained consultants were available. Initially two Macmillan nurses were also appointed. The Health Authority intended that the Pembridge Unit should provide a service for Paddington, North Kensington and Brent, with the understanding that in due course the facilities would be transferred to St. Charles' Hospital, Ladbroke Grove, as a component of the proposed Community Hospital.

When the Pembridge Unit opened in the Harrow Road, 24 beds were transferred from Hereford and Chepstow Lodges to the same site to form the community unit, and 19 to St. Charles' Hospital to form a rehabilitation unit in the upgraded Nightingale Ward. The community unit was subsequently closed for financial reasons. The occupancy was unsatisfactory, making revenue expenditure unduly high, and therefore the future for the

Community Hospital is problematical (in 1991). The continuing care and hospice beds remain and are well used.

Sexually-transmitted diseases

Paddington appeared to attract substantial numbers of men of all ages suffering from sexually-transmitted diseases, and great pride was taken in the level of excellence and caring provided in the Special Clinic on Praed Street with its associated beds for in-patients. As the incidence of AIDS increased and with it greater public awareness and anxiety, St. Mary's Hospital under the leadership of Dr. Anthony Pinching and Dr. 'Willy' Harris and their colleagues, was foremost in the field of care and education regarding the risks of unprotected sex and multiple sexual partnerships. The Jefferies Research Wing was opened in June, 1983, by Sir Christopher Booth, then Director, Clinical Research Centre, Northwick Park Hospital (Medical Research Council).

Concurrent to increased awareness of the medical and social tragedy of AIDS came the marked increase in drug dependency, heroin being the hard drug favoured at the time.

The Authority in an endeavour to meet this challenge, established a 'walk in' drug dependency unit in a prefabricated building adjacent to the District Offices. An adjoining caravan housed the needle exchange service. The nursing staff and the staff of the District Psychology Service, through work in these various facilities, built up a national reputation in counselling patients with AIDS and related illnesses, and have taken a major part in training staff in other parts of the country.

Mental illness services

When in October, 1983, the Woodfield Wing closed for renovation at Harrow Road, the Paterson Wing on the canal site was opened, providing accommodation for 60 in-patients with acute mental illness and 80 day hospital places. In 1985, a further two units were opened at St. Charles' Hospital, to provide accommodation for the elderly with acute mental illness and with dementias respectively. In part the two units were to house patients formerly cared for at Banstead Hospital in Surrey so that they would now reside within their own home districts. The day hospital care was naturally integral to the services for the mentally ill.

Dr. Mark Arden was appointed early in 1985 as Consultant in the Psychiatry of Old Age, and Professor Bruce Pitt in 1986 to the Professorship in the same subject. Both appointments greatly enhanced the services provided to the elderly in the District. A daily case conference considered the needs of all new patients seen in the preceding 24 hours. The emphasis was placed by the senior staff in all of the contributing health care disciplines, on maintaining people in their own homes as long as possible, and admission to hospital as an in-patient was kept to a minimum, except for assessment purposes. Four years later a similar policy was enshrined in legislation.

Sick children

The physical and psychiatric treatment of sick children was debated at great length. Acute services initially were provided at Paddington Green Children's Hospital, at St. Mary's Hospital, Praed Street, and at St. Charles' Hospital. Paddington Green was used largely in support of children with chronic or intercurrent disease such as *thallasaemia* and *sickle cell anaemia*, and those with permanent disabilities. The District Disability Team was based there, providing domiciliary care, and as such was a pre-cursor to 'care in the community'.

Despite its cramped and out-dated circumstances, Peter Pan Ward at St. Charles' Hospital was greatly prized by the local population, serving as it did the socially deprived area of North Kensington. The Authority embarked upon substantial upgrading of this ward to provide fewer but more suitable bed-spaces and facilities. A specialised paediatric casualty department and a 'walk in' service available to parents and others, set the scene for subsequent developments toward a Community Hospital based at St. Charles' Hospital.

In due course when the Queen Elizabeth the Queen Mother Wing on South Wharf Road was opened, all acute childrens' services were centralised, including those at St. Charles' Hospital and Paddington Green Children's Hospital. The latter was closed, and the beautiful tiles depicting classical fairy tales were saved and transferred to the new wards.

Children's psychiatric services were liberally provided across the District, based in various centres including Paddington Green and North Kensington. There was a perceived over-provision and a lack of coherence despite much   invaluable and dedicated work in this field, but these problems have proved difficult to rectify.

Adults with learning difficulties

Services for adults with learning difficulties were provided jointly between Westminster City Council and the District Health Authority. A small purpose-built unit, comprising two bungalows, was based on a site adjacent to the (then) St. Mary's Hospital, Harrow Road, with frontage onto the Harrow Road itself. This unit, owing much to Dr. John Dunwoody and his staff, particularly Dr. William Kearns, was the first of its kind in inner London. In-patient, respite and out-patient day care was offered to clients, and served as a model pattern of care for the future.

Achievements at St. Mary's*

During these years much remarkable research and development was underway both in academic and service departments of St. Mary's and its associated hospitals: A new academic Department of Cardiology was created. Professor Desmond Sheridan was appointed to the Chair in 1985, and Dr. Rodney Foale joined the staff as Consultant Cardiologist. Work on genetic abnormality and disease, notably that being undertaken by Professor Bob Williamson in conjunction with researchers in Copenhagen, Toronto and Salt Lake City on the gene responsible for cystic fibrosis, was immensely exciting both to scientists and, even more so, to families at risk.

The skill and leadership of Mr. Harry Eastcott in the field of vascular surgery was widely acknowledged throughout the world. We were fortunate indeed in recruiting Avril Mansfield as his successor. Her modesty and charm in addition to her undoubted talent was and remains a joy to the hospital and to her many friends.

*   Politics of Progress, by Ewan Ferlie & Andrew Pettigrew, **Health Services Journal,** 12.1.89

The Department of Renal Medicine, including the Dialysis Unit was housed in pre-war accommodation and approached by a somewhat unreliable lift at the top of a ramp formerly used by horses employed by British Rail on the Great Western Railway. The indefatigable Drs. Barry Hulme and Roger Gabriel, Consultants in charge of the Unit, once told me as I ascended the ramp on my way to the Treasurer's Department, that the ability to mount this ramp provided valuable evidence of a patient's suitability for transplant.

In anticipation of the Queen Elizabeth the Queen Mother Wing, Dr. Oscar Craig and his colleagues enthusiastically pursued the latest in technological developments in the Department of Radiology. This included digital substraction angiography, a computerised system producing clear images and substracting unwanted features of an image or highlighting areas of importance under investigation - of great value in cardiac and vascular angiography. Dr. Craig's careful explanation to me of the advantages of these developments and the relevance to the work of the Departments of Cardiology and Vascular Surgery (among others) gave me immense pleasure, insofar as any contribution I might be able to make in support of both.

Dr. Hugh Baron's work in gastro-enterology and his contribution as a member of the Health Authority was highly valued by those who worked with him, as was that of his colleague David Paintin, Reader in Obstetrics and Gynaecology, a deeply thoughtful and caring surgeon. Hugh Baron's interest alongside medicine was the use of many forms of art in hospitals. He exercised substantial national influence in this sphere and locally encouraged the liberal use of tapestries and pictorial art in the Queen Elizabeth the Queen Mother Wing, retaining the artist Bridget Riley as advisor. Hugh was largely responsible for an imaginative series of murals in the Peter Pan Children's Unit at St. Charles' Hospital as executed by the artist Stephen Selwyn.

Mother and Baby Care

The Maternity Unit and the Winnicot Baby Unit were housed in extremely cramped conditions at St. Mary's Hospital. It was imperative that both should be upgraded. The suggestion that maternity services should be provided on two sites - namely, St. Mary's Harrow Road and at Praed Street, or alternatively based only at Harrow Road was fiercely contested. For a combination of good reasons, it was decided to base the in-patient care at Praed Street, and some additional ante-natal, out-patient services on the ground floor of the newly upgraded Woodfield Wing, Harrow Road - convenient to expectant mothers from that locality. I was delighted to open the new unit in October 1984.

The importance of the Birthright Centre under the Patronage of HRH The Princess of Wales, which was jointly funded by the Philip and Pauline Harris Charitable Trust and 'Birthright', cannot be overstated.

Research into recurrent miscarriage in pregnancy resulting from immunological incompatability between mother's and child's systems, and the treatment of selected sufferers, was pursued by Professor Beard, Professor Mowbray and their colleagues. The painstaking efforts made by this team, turning tragedy to delight for countless parents, are recorded in a gallery of photographs of the babies successfully delivered.

A forward-looking midwifery staff under the influence of Joan Greenwood followed by Liz MacAnulty and the leadership of Professor Richard Beard, Sir George Pinker, Alisdair Fraser, Frank Leoffler and colleagues, ensured the high reputation of St. Mary's in the obstetrics field, as does the on-going work supported by St. Mary's 'Save the Baby Fund' and its five major projects.

Royalty and St. Mary's...

St. Mary's Hospital and the Medical School have long enjoyed the interest and support of members of the Royal Family. Queen Elizabeth the Queen Mother visited the School of Nursing on several occasions during the years about which I write, and laid the Foundation Stone in 1983, of the new building which bears her name.

Much to the delight of all concerned, she later performed the Opening Ceremony. Thus the Queen Mother continued the tradition as in June, 1931 when Duchess of York, she had laid the foundation stone of the new medical school. In June, 1845, Prince Albert, Consort of Queen Victoria, laid the Foundation stone of what was originally known as the Paddington and Marylebone Hospital, later known as St. Mary's (due, it is said, to the proximity of St. Mary's Church and the gift of the land by the Bishop of London.)

On the 27th February, 1985, on the occasion of the formal opening, the Health District was honoured by the visit of HM The Queen and HRH The Duke of Edinburgh to the Queen's Park Health Centre. Their visit greatly encouraged those who live and work in this deprived part of North Kensington.

HRH the Princess Royal visited the Medical School in order to lay the Foundation Stone of the Students Sport Centre at Wilson House.

HRH the Princess of Wales, in addition to entrusting herself to the Lindo Wing for the birth of her two sons, has tirelessly supported 'Birthright' as Patron, and has also shown great interest in the aims of the 'Save the Baby Fund'. She is equally committed to the work of the hospital in care of patients with AIDS.

The Friends of St. Mary's were fortunate that Lady Jane Fellowes became Patron of that organisation and subsequently has shown unflagging interest and support for their work.

... And moments of sadness

As in all histories, St. Mary's experienced tragedies along with the joys. In July, 1982, soldiers injured in the Regents Park bombing incident, following on from the appalling slaughter of soldiers and horses in Hyde Park, were admitted to St. Mary's Hospital. Under circumstances which would have daunted many, the staff responded magnificently to this devastating event. The Accident and Emergency Department in the 'old' St. Mary's was cramped and inconvenient, as was the Intensive Care Unit. None were prepared for the sight of such dreadful injuries as those sustained by these young soldiers, all bandsmen of the Royal Green Jackets. The Green Jackets gave a charity concert at the Royal Albert Hall in July, 1983, and it was wonderful that many of the injured musicians were then able to play to a packed house. A most moving tribute was given by Sir Roger Bannister.

The Chairman, Members and Staff
of Paddington and North Kensington
Health Authority are deeply honoured
and delighted in that The Heir
Apparent to the Throne as Head of
the Commonwealth and Dependencies
Overseas was born in St Mary's
Hospital, Praed Street on 21 June 1982

WE send our loyal and affectionate
congratulations and greetings
and we wish the baby PRINCE
and his parents their
ROYAL HIGHNESSES THE
PRINCE AND PRINCESS
OF WALES a long and happy
life together in peace, good health
and freedom.

St Mary's Hospital
Praed Street
Paddington
London W2

Chapter 15
The Medical Research Council

Appointment to the Medical Research Council (MRC) is afforded to few lay members, and as one of two such serving from 1979 through 1987, it was personally of immense interest and pleasure. For this privilege I am especially grateful to Sir Keith Joseph, then Secretary of State for Education and Science, for both my first and second terms of office, at such a momentous period in the history of medical research. Medical science is always exciting, but perhaps in these years even more so as prominent ethical issues emerged related to in-vitro fertilisation, and research into genetic defects using human embryos.

The Report of the Department of Health and Social Security Committee of Inquiry into Human Fertilisation and Embryology, known as the *Warnock Report (Cmd 9314)* was considered by the MRC in December, 1984. Their considered response was informed by the work of the Advisory Group set up to review Policy on Research on In-vitro Fertilisation (Chairman: Professor G.S. Dawes, FRS). Subsequently, the matter was debated in the House of Commons, the Private

Members Bill introduced by Mr. Enoch Powell failing through lack of parliamentary time.

The potential results for humanity of genetic engineering were immeasurable, and clearly demanded strict controls. To that end a Government-sponsored committee, independent of the MRC, was formed under the chairmanship of Baroness Warnock. Research units engaged in embryo research were monitored closely, and experimentation on the human embryo beyond fourteen days gestation prohibited. Cross-species fertilisation, employed in research into human sub-fertility required careful explanation, and this was given through the MRC's *Annual Report* to Parliament. Naturally many aspects of this work, such as the use of frozen embryos, the use of frozen sperm deposited before death and other equally challenging scientific possibilities, require on-going debate and great wisdom. The House of Commons finally debated some of these matters on 23rd April, 1990, and the results are embodied in the *Human Fertilisation and Embryology Bill (1990)*.

Another subject of medical responsibility which was long studied and debated during my tenure, was the MRC Vitamin Study. This project was set up in response to a request for advice from the Health Department about the role of vitamin supplementation in general, and the use of vitamins in *Pregnavite Forte F* in particular, in the prevention of spina bifida and anencephalic births among women who had already experienced one such birth. Further research was required before clinical practice advice could be given, and therefore a multi-centre controlled trial was proposed with 29 centres in five countries taking part. Exercising the Council was the possible need to stop the study if clear evidence of the efficacy of vitamins in preventing neural tube defects was to emerge; it would no longer then be defensible to withold the vitamins from the control group.

The use of animals in medical research was then, as now, a subject giving rise to much controversy - and occasional demonstrations and picketting of MRC Units. The *Animals (Scientific Procedures) Bill* was published and received its first reading in the House of Lords on 14th November, 1985.

During my time on the MRC, I chaired the Committee's Standing Committee to update its statement on *Responsibility in the use of medical information for research: Principles and Guide to Practice*. The work extended over many months and upon occasion feelings ran high between members. Some were fearful lest undue restrictions and controls would jeopardise the work of clinical researchers while others feared that undue licence would endanger the confidential relationship between doctors and patients. After long negotiation, the MRC Statement was issued in 1985.

A major privilege afforded to serving MRC members was the opportunity to meet and listen to erudite and learned medical scientists from all over the world. I had never expected to meet Nobel Prize winners, still less had I expected the modesty of these great men and women who went to untold lengths to explain in simpler terms the intricacies of their work. Their skills and humility were made even more obvious by their efforts to be clear and understandable.

In 1987 a meeting to celebrate the 40th birthday of molecular biology was held at the Cavendish Laboratory in Cambridge. The invited guests - among whom I was one - listened to some of the original participants in the work, including Max Perutz, Francis Crick and Cesar Milstein [the winner of the Nobel Prize for work on monoclonal antibodies].

Then as now, financial stringency in relation to research, and development of findings was uppermost in the minds of those required to judge applications to the MRC for financial support. Whether concerning a project grant, or the institution of an entire research unit, anxieties were evidenced about the threat of commercialism overtaking the pursuit of scientific knowledge as an end it itself. Illustration of these worries is found in a leading article published in 1987, and is reprinted here. It describes our concerns more graphically than I can.

Bicycle sheds make imperfect laboratories. But, if the money's there to pay for people, heating and equipment, few scientists would complain. Give them some hope that one day there could be a spanking new laboratory and you have the makings of a world famous institution. This is just what happened when the Medical Research Council's Laboratory of Molecular Biology was born in Cambridge.

As several of the scientists present in those early days of molecular biology point out in this issue of New Scientist, the last thing that concerned them when they were trying to unravel the chemistry of life was the cost of doing it. Today the ever-present fear for many scientists, if not those working at the Laboratory of Molecular Biology, must be that the institution they work for will be forced to sell off the by now slightly seedy and run-down laboratory to a property speculator, while the researchers move back into the bike shed. (Actually this ploy wouldn't work because the government would confiscate the 'profits' from any property speculation).

Next to last in the thinking of the people who went on to win seven Nobel prizes was the money that their research would make for their paymasters, let alone themselves. At the time, the scientists in Cambridge had little thought for the 'use' of their work. They were doing it to advance knowledge. Working as they were at the frontiers of biology, they clearly hoped to learn something about the basic process of life. Such knowledge would inevitably have consequences for medical research in the long term, but there was no thought of 'wonder drugs' and the like. Today every scientist who receives so much as the cost of a postage stamp from the public purse has to think of short-term ways of recovering the taxpayers' outlay.

Of course, there was 'spinoff' from the work at Cambridge, perhaps the most famous being the development that won Cesar Milstein his Nobel Prize for monoclonal antibodies. The Laboratory of Molecular Biology is seen as the home of at least one lost opportunity. When Milstein worked out how to produce cell lines that create a single type of antibody, he was more interested in solving a scientific problem that in making money for his laboratory or for British industry. The laboratory did suggest that there might just possibly be some commercial mileage in Milstein's work, but the body that was supposed to protect the 'intellectual property' amassed by government-funded R & D declined the offer.

Too many people have bemoaned this failure to patent and to exploit this important breathrough - one of the companies around the world, especially in the United States, have developed to their own benefit. The mood of the time was right. Scientists shouldn't be rummaging around looking for every penny they can bring in. Milstein's idea rightly belonged to the world. It is not the fault of anyone at Cambridge that British industry failed to realise how ubiquitous the monoclonal antibody would become. (Actually it is wrong to suggest that British companies missed the boat with monoclonal antibodies; ask Amersham International, to name just one. Where it would be today without these important biological tools?) No one has kept count, but the laboratory in Cambridge must have paid for itself many times over in its 40 years. And while extremists in the scientific community are wrong to reject any contact with the sordid 'real world' it is equally wrong that many scientists now have to scramble around trying to justify their research by promising short-term returns.

Such is the pressure from the paymasters - and the acquiescence of the paid - that the day is far too near when straightforward scientific advances, as opposed to commercial developments, will push up the price of shares in some company or other. There they are, trying to patent well-known materials that have suddenly revealed themselves to be super-conductors, not to mention 'life forms' that just might have some commercial use. It won't be long before any one discovers the modern equivalent of the notion that salt makes chips more tasty, or that sperm fertilise eggs, will rush to apply for a patent.

This 'mercantile' tendency" may be an especially British one - after all, scientists in this country who want to stay in business have every reason to scramble around in the dirt in search of an excuse to ask for more money - but the message is depressingly international. You couldn't set up a laboratory that gave 'shed room' to the likes of Max Perutz, Aaron Klug, James Watson, Francis Crick, Cesar Milstein, Fred Sanger, Hugh Huxley, John Kendrew and so on unless they guaranteed to deliver marketable ideas, molecules and organisms that one of the already wealthy members of the pharmaceutical industry could turn into greater profit.

Perhaps though, 'oddballs' like those who gave birth to molecular biology would not find lab space today, not even in the bicycle shed. One MRC Committee met last week and shortage of money forced it to reject at least two-thirds of the research projects that it considered to be worthwhile. Even if the committee had been able to find the money, some of the research teams would have been hobbled by a shortage of staff because the bright young scientists who would have done the work, the 'post docs' who would expect to spend a few years working on short-term contracts, will no longer accept the risk of being left permanently in this twilight zone between being a student and a full-time member of the scientific profession.

Forty years on and science has changed out of all recognition. Today, the only laboratories that can hope to win a steady flow of Nobel prizes are run by multinational corporations whose R & D budgets dwarf those of many countries. It is no accident that IBM, AT&T and similarly wealthy corporations are taking over from the likes of Cambridge in the Nobel stakes. This makes the achievements of the Laboratory of Molecular Biology even more remarkable. Let us hope that the laboratory will still be there to celebrate a 50th birthday, let alone an 80th.

New Scientist, 21 May, 1987, **London**

Chapter 16
Restructuring and Reorganisation in the NHS

1972-3, 1981-2, 1989-90

The pattern and prevalence of illness and disease has changed significantly in this century. Thinking back to between the wars and then proceeding forward in thought from the inception of the National Health Service, many infectious diseases and disabling conditions are virtually unknown today. While rejoicing in the conquest of such horrors as diptheria, scarlet fever, poliomyelitis, the NHS nevertheless finds itself embattled. A continuous struggle rages for necessary resources - human and financial - with which to confront and contain demands resulting from demographic changes and advances in medical science and technology.

Rapid medical developments and genuine progress in the delivery of medical care have resulted in unprecedented expectations and demands from previously silent and passive recipients of health services. Vascular surgery, transplant surgery, curative treatment of previously fatal diseases, survival of very low birth-weight and premature infants, increased understanding of obscure medical problems, and early diagnosis of potentially life-threatening conditions all lead to increased longevity. While the population of disabled, handicapped, and elderly dependent people increases -people who can function well in their own environments if helped appropriately - a constant escalation of costs occurs in the NHS and social support services and the number of active, wage-earners and tax-payers decreases.

That part of the gross national product committed to the NHS is a matter of constant comment and debate, as is comparison with other so-called advanced nations. It is certain that with today's medical practice and in light of future developments, demands will be infinite. Resources will just as certainly be finite and dependant upon the corporate wealth of the United Kingdom.

In the early 1960s the NHS in management terms was little more than a cottage industry. Now there is widespread acknowledgement that the changes detailed above place increasing demands upon the service and require both a style of management and a level of sophistication not required in earlier years. And when currently one hears vociferous demands on the part of the medical profession to preserve the status quo, it is well to recollect the opposition to the concept of a national health service from the same quarters in the 1940s.

Serious students of NHS history will find what they require in textbooks elsewhere. Since this is a volume of 'snapshots' only a brief summary of reports and legislation is included here. The latter half of the 1960s provided a harvest of rationalising and restructuring documents begun perhaps by the appearance of the *Farquharson Lang Report (Report on Administrative Practice of Hospital Boards in Scotland - 1966)* which made sweeping recommendations for the role and function of Board members, and contained major implications for the NHS in England. Also, in 1966, the *Salmon Committee (Report on the Career Structure for Senior Nursing Staff)* presented its recommendations, introducing a grading system for 'nurse managers'. In addition the *Cogwheel Report (Report on the Organisation of Medical* Work *in Hospital)* in 1967 presaged substantial if not radical changes in the pattern and style of NHS management.

Two Green Papers on NHS structure were published respectively in 1968 *(NHS: The Administrative Structure of the Medical and Related Services in England & Wales)* and in 1970 *(NHS: The Future Structure of the National Health Service in England)*. In 1971 a consultative document followed these up *(NHS Reorganisation Consultative Document)* and then in 1972 the *NHS Command Paper 5055 (NHS Reorganisation: England - August; Management Arrangements for the Reorganised*

NHS - September) completed the documentation. A major theme throughout this work was the need to lessen the professional isolation felt by those working in hospitals for the mentally ill and mentally handicapped, to remove the stigma of working with and suffering from such conditions, and to ensure economies of scale within the NHS as a whole.

The underlying philosophy of the 1972 re-organisation (as generated by McKinsey consultants through their 'Grey Book' advice) was in the concept of consensus management through which senior staff from all departments would play an active part in managing the Service. Initially this was welcomed by professional staff of all disciplines. The creation of teams of officers at Regional, Area and District levels, including administrators, doctors, dentists, nurses, finance and works officers, and the appointment of District Officers in disciplines such as catering, pharmacy, radiology, occupational therapy and others, publicly acknowledged the importance of many skills in the totality of patient care.

Concurrent with management re-organisation in hospital services came the attempt to integrate fully the Family Doctor services into mainstream NHS administration. Similarly the majority of public health services - District Nurses, Health Visitors, District Midwives and School Health workers - were transferred from the responsibility of Local Authorities to the NHS. 'Hospital almoners' became 'hospital social workers' and thereby employees of the Local Authorities, to the dismay of some professional staff and Health Authorities.

At the time of these multiple changes I remained Chairman of the HMC in Cornwall, while 'shadowing' the Chairmanship of the new Health Authority. Therefore I was charged with the responsibility for setting up the new Authority and appointing Members to the Family Practitioner Committee (FPC) which replaced the Executive Council. No senior staff were available to assist me in this task; a retired Administrator visited at monthly intervals during the six month lead-in period.

The method set up for appointing senior staff - and especially the Area Administrators across the country - was a complex 'matching' process, whereby the wishes of the applicants were matched with the recommendations of the Authorities. Thus the applicant would list his preferences as between the Authorities where he had been shortlisted; these would be matched with those of the interviewing committees. If the first match was impossible, second or third choices would be offered. Of itself, the method in some instances proved both distressing and invidious, and led to confidentiality being breached more often than observed.

An account of Cornish health services at that time and in the years that followed during my Chairmanship would be incomplete without reference to the enthusiastic work of the Area team of officers. They sought corporately and individually to guide the Authority toward new management concepts at a time of rapid changes, industrial unrest, and strong Trade Union influence. In Dr. Harry Binysh and later Dr. Peter Gentle, Cornwall found the beneficial influence of Medical Officers of high intelligence and unfailing courtesy. Donald Swift proved a worthy successor to John Green, having qualities of leadership and determination to achieve and maintain the highest standards of nursing care. Gerry Roberts' abilities and 'wizardry' as a Treasurer were renowned - and not only in the South West Region. Firm financial management never seemed to preclude, if on occasion by what seemed a miracle, the necessary monetary support for a valuable scheme.

In Alan Hodder the Authority was most fortunate to find an Administrator of great ability, determination and integrity. I was aware of his personal attributes through knowing of his work as Deputy to Harold White at the South West Regional Hospital Board. I had hoped to attract him to Cornwall during the matching process described above, and I was delighted when we were successful.

Reorganisation and its failures

The 1972 re-organisation so hopefully embarked upon nevertheless failed in a number of aspects. Three tiers of management were cumbersome and costly. Accountability was ill defined and responsibility obscured. Whereas Regional and Area teams of officers had clearly prescribed duties for which they were severally responsible to the Authority, the Administrator was perceived by the general public and by medical staff as 'first among equals.' Members were appointed to Area and Regional Authorities but played no immediate part at District level. The mangement of services in hospitals was highly unsatisfactory in one telling respect close to the heart of many: the highly valued personage, the 'Matron' who was recognised by all as an authority figure, was replaced by a 'nursing officer' at the top of a numbered scale. Imagine a 'Matron', no, imagine a '9' or a '10'! This had been the work of the Salmon Committee, and proved very unpopular. Further, the intention to integrate the Family Doctor services more closely with those of the hospital services was not realised.

Increasingly, concerns were voiced about the health and welfare of the NHS at Government level and in the country at large. A Royal Commission was appointed to investigate the whole arena of problems, and a report emerged in July,

1979. A final chapter, issued separately, was entitled *A Service for Patients*. Publication of the whole of the Royal Commission Report was rapidly followed by *Patients First (Consultative Paper on the Structure and Management of the NHS in England and Wales)* published in December, 1979. Thus, in 1981, the Government embarked on yet another change. Single district Areas became District Health Authorities and multi-district Areas were divided into autonomous District Authorities, the Area Authorities ceasing to exist. Once more senior officers were obliged to enter the job market in search of a post concomitant with their seniority and experience. Many had already re-applied for their existing post upon the integration of General and Psychiatric/Mental Handicap HMCs, and again at the time of the 1972 re-organisation.

In 1983 the Service was again confronted by a major change in the form of the *Griffiths Report (Part I: NHS Management Enquiry, October, 1983)*. This Report, based on a study by Roy Griffiths (later Sir) recommended a change in management structure from that of a team of officers of roughly equal seniority - the Administrator as 'first amongst equals' - to that of a structure headed up by a General Manager. The latter's role would comprise broadly the duties and responsibilities of a manager in commerce and industry as well as those generally understood to accrue to the health service post. Contracts should be limited to a period of three years, subject to performance review, and to be renewable if mutually satisfactory. Holders of the General Managerial posts would relinquish their rights under the Employment Protection legislation.

Paddington and North Kensington Health Authority accepted the Griffiths recommendations as reasonable and in the interests of the NHS. They recommended their current Administrator to the post of General Manager. Inadvertently that recommendation was put forward as a foregone conclusion, and a question was raised in Parliament about the Authority setting precedents in advance of the necessary regulations. In fact, the position was regularised in due course, and the appointment of the District Administrator, Terry Hunt in this instance, to the post of District General Manager was duly confirmed.

Terry Hunt gained rapid promotion and within a few months was appointed Regional General Manager to the South East Thames RHA. Thus the Authority embarked again in 1985 on the managerial changes which other authorities were experiencing, and appointed Barbara Young, a foremost and energetic young General Manager.

Subsequent to the implementation of Griffiths, there was an increasing recognition of the complexity and high cost of health services. Taken in conjunction with Conservative government policies - under Mrs. Thatcher's leadership - the end result was two White Papers: *Working for Patients,* covering hospital services, and *Caring for People* to cover the care of people in the community. The latter followed in broad terms many of the Griffiths recommendations as contained in *Community Care - Agenda for Action* (Part II, March 1988) which in turn had followed the publication of the Audit Commission for Local Authorities in England and Wales entitled, *Making a Reality of Community Care.*

What do the proposed changes in management structure mean? It is hoped and expected that a new style of leadership more closely related to industry will emerge. The smaller Management Boards, comprising both Executive and non-Executive Directors should lead to an efficient, cost-effective service. The care of elderly and disabled people, the mentally ill and those with learning difficulties, are to be assisted primarily under the aegis of the Local Authorities. With the role of Health Authorities being that of 'purchasers' of services rather than 'providers' - from independent Trusts or from directly managed units - a new level of expertise and sophistication will be required.

In 1990 responsibility for health policy was vested in the Policy Board under the Chairmanship of the Secretary of State, and implementation of policy delegated to the Management Executive under the Chairmanship of the NHS Chief Executive. Newly appointed Boards of Executive and non-Executive Directors at District and Trust level are in process of establishing their status and authority vis-a-vis the 'centre'. It is anticipated that Community Health Councils will continue in their roles to safeguard the public, although District Authorities are exhorted to regard themselves as 'Champions of the public'. Concurrently, far reaching developments in the management of family doctor services are also proposed, as a result of two Command papers issued in April 1986 (*Primary Health Care)* and November 1987 *(Improving Primary Health Care*) respectively.

Family Practitioner Committees have become the Family Health Service Authorities, managed similarly to the hospital services by small Boards of Directors with professional and lay members. The contracts of medical and dental practitioners are to be more tightly controlled, and medical practitioners in large practices to be encouraged to "manage" their own budgets.

In January, 1988, many Authorities reviewed their priorities in relation to preventive medicine and the control of communicable diseases as a result of the publication of *Public Health in England*. The important role of public health doctors was emphasized and new appointments of high calibre medical staff were made to these departments. Project 2000 is projected to introduce substantial changes in the preparation of nurses to staff hospital and community services, and for those colleges of nursing studies where contracts have been placed for the new training pro-grammes, dramatic re-organisation and re-structuring has already taken place.

The National Health Service is again subjected to fundamental change, causing anxiety in some quarters to staff and patients alike, and in others a sense of challenge and optimism. Nevertheless, I perceive a deeply rooted determination on the part of professional staff I meet - in all disciplines - that they will remain unfailingly dedicated as in years past, to the service of their patients.

Chapter 17
Chairmanship: pleasures, perils and pitfalls

"Up the airy mountain, down the rushy glen" with apologies to   William Allingham (1828 - 1889)

As the Health Service has changed and, in real terms, increased in complexity and cost, so the level of answerability to the taxpayer through Parliament has become more immediate. The practice of medicine and the management of the service is now conducted in the public arena, subject to scrutiny and to comment, politically sensitive and demanding of sophisticated financial and general management.

The personal traits evident in the majority of Management Committee chairmen in the 1960s and early 1970s differ somewhat from those exhibited in later appointments in successive re-organisations. Most chairmen had served previously as Committee members, and had committed themselves to the NHS to the exclusion of other absorbing, outside interests. Many were self-employed in managing family businesses. Preponderantly from professional backgrounds, party political allegiance was never mentioned and tainly not evident. The NHS was far from being the'political football' it has become in later years.

The Chairman was expected by all staff - professional or supporting - to give time and interest to many and varied social occasions throughout the year. At Christmas every unit would be visited by the Chairman and the Group Secretary (the General Manager of these days). The Regional Hospital Board expected the Chairman to visit every hospital at regular intervals, and to acquire and maintain an intimate knowledge of the services provided. In the aftermath of the 'Sans Everything' enquiries, these visits were regarded as overriding responsibility in hospitals for the mentally ill and mentally handicapped.

The Chairman of the South Western Regional Hospital Board, John English, expressed the hope that all Chairmen would know our staff by name. This was something of a tall order from the perspective of the Cornwall Hospital Management Committee which employed some 6000 people - but I would endeavour to learn the names of all we would meet during any visit he made, from senior medical staff to porter. In reality as Chairman of Cornwall for 10 years I knew by name a great number of staff at all levels. Most Chairmen also regarded it as important to visit the hospitals at night, especially those for the mentally ill and mentally handicapped as the effort was richly repaid in learning more of the conditions under which staff were working and patients were living.

In those days the Chairman of the HMC was expected to play an important role in public life and public relations, to be on friendly terms with Chairmen and Mayors of Local Authorities, and to attend such occasions as 'Mayor Making' in the various cities and towns served by the hospitals. The Chairman would be invited to other civic ceremonies as well, and regular meetings with Members of Parliament were encouraged.

In the years prior to the *Farquharson-Lang Report (1966)* as already referred, committee and sub-committee work had proliferated to an unacceptable level. Nevertheless, for those of us unversed in estate management and the intricacies of electrical and mechanical engineering, the kind of 'tutoring' provided by committee work was instructive and valuable. Prior to the integration of the General Group in Cornwall with that of St. Lawrence and Associated Hospitals the demands upon my time as Chairman were entirely compatible with that of the part-time post held with Cornwall County Council.

Over these years it became increasingly evident that the Group Secretary (executive administrator) role needed to change, to resemble that of a manager in commerce or industry. That change would require a corresponding change in the role of Chairman - from any semblance of an executive position toward that of a non-executive Chairman or figurehead. The 1972-3 re-organisation reinforced and expedited these changes, requiring great efforts not only to change the spots on the leopard but to be seen to do so.

Difficulties, both apparent and real, were exacerbated in Cornwall. Notwithstanding the personal friendship and sustained and mutual effort between the Area Administrator and myself to reach a satisfactory working relationship, I could see that senior staff loyalties were stretched and divided. Reluctantly I concluded that I had failed to change my leadership style sufficiently to fit the new role, and decided to resign at the close of my first term of office as Chairman for the Cornwall and Isles of Scilly Area Health Authority.

Accordingly in 1977 I wrote to the Secretary of State indicating that as I had served for ten years as Chairman in Cornwall, I felt that it would not be in the best interest of the service for me to continue in that role. My resignation was accepted. I received great support at this difficult time from the Permanent Secretary to the Department, Sir Patrick Nairne, and the Deputy Secretary, James Collier, to both of whom I owe unremitting gratitude.

On being appointed Chairman of Paddington and North Kensington Health Authority in 1981, my determination to avoid any resemblance to an Executive Chairman, approached a level of paranoia. Two totally unconnected factors helped me to resist any temptations otherwise. Firstly, I had by then experienced the professional frustration and difficulty of working as Director to a charitable trust under an Executive Chairman - albeit of great charm and ability. Secondly, I was now working with a District Administrator who had worked in the District for a number of years which was quite the reverse of the situation I had left in Cornwall. I was now the 'outsider', the unknown quantity in the equation. Both with the District Administrator and later with his successor, Barbara Young, I was able to talk through my fears of usurping the role that was theirs. Inevitably there were occasions which caused us mutual anxieties but frank discussion rapidly resolved any potential rift which arose.

The importance of Vice-Chairmen during these years cannot be exaggerated. The support, guidance and loyalty shown to me by successive vice-chairmen far exceeded all that any Chairman might reasonably expect. In Cornwall, Captain Andy Palmer and the late Leslie Northey both restrained and encouraged me through very testing times (which included written threats to my life and the menaces of the occult). In Paddington and North Kensington, Joe Bennett and David Paintin, Reader in obstetrics and gynaecology at St. Mary's Hospital Medical School were equally wise and supportive - although the threats amounted to no more than verbal abuse and the odd soft, harmless missile.

Appearance before a Select Committee of the House of Commons provided insights into the democratic machinery of Government and how the ultimate rights of aggrieved citizens are upheld. In this instance, the Health Parliamentary Commissioner for Administration (the Ombudsman) in the course of his customary scrutiny of cases, had selected a complaint related to St. Mary's Hospital, Paddington. Mr. Anthony Barrowclough, then the Commissioner, had decided that this particular complaint warranted a personal explanation, and I was summoned along with Barbara Young, the General Manager, to appear before the All Party Select Committee.

Searching questions were put to us and evidence was collected and explored in every respect. We recounted the sad circumstances surrounding the particular death, and were treated with great courtesy and understanding. I came away with great respect for the Members' intentions to discover the truth in the interest of the individual patient and his relatives. Nevertheless, to appear before a Select Committee is a salutory experience, and one striking example of the vicarious responsibility carried by chairmen and general managers even though they play no direct part in the circumstances of the particular event.

1991 Forward

*Management is management.......is management
.......or is it?*

Frequently it is alleged that qualities required
in managing a major industrial concern or indeed
a chain of grocery stores, are not necessarily those
which are appropriate to chairmen and managers
of health services. Clearly a total commitment to
the NHS and to the care of patients and their
health needs is an absolute must. Without that
commitment the necessary and enthusiastic
leadership would be difficult if not impossible to
display with conviction. With this proviso, it is now
evident that a high level of competence and sophisticated management skills are vital components
for success. The technology and art of medicine,
escalating costs, competing demands upon the
public purse, and the demands of a newly struc-
tured bureaucracy all require expertise.

In 1991, therefore, any chairman will require
additional qualities to those possessed by chairmen appointed in previous decades. Authorities
have been transformed into small management
boards of executive and non-executive directors.
The role is to become one of 'purchasing' and
monitoring rather than 'providing' services. The
relationship, as it evolves between DHAs, RHAs,

and the independent NHS Trusts is one which will be watched and studied with interest. Equally the evolving role of the FHSAs will elicit the same scrutiny. The latter are regarded by some as de facto Primary Health Care Authorities and by others as likely to subsume the role of District Authorities.

Whatever management structure ultimately emerges, the need will remain for a relationship of trust and loyalty between chairman and 'General Manager' (whatever title is used), and the senior directors. The Chairman will as in the past be required to exert and to display qualities of leadership in gaining the confidence of members of the Board and of the staff working within the organisation. It is well to remember that however comprehensive the changes in the overall NHS structure, professional staff of all the disciplines involved will remain the means whereby care is delivered to patients who are after all our clients and customers.

It is hoped that in future the difficulties and uncertainties experienced by me and many colleagues, whereby as chairmen we carried ultimate responsibility without clear executive authority, have been swept away, and replaced by a management structure more appropriate to the needs of a highly complex health service. Dual loyalty and responsibility to the public on the one hand and to the Secretary of State on the other, in whose gift lies the appointments of chairmen, will continue upon occasion to create tension and self doubt. Such doubts can only be resolved by certainty as to the commitment of government, of whatever persuasion, to support an efficient and caring health service.

Having served under many Secretaries and Ministers of State, both Labour and Conservative, I have not experienced any such doubts. Had I done so, I would certainly have resigned. As it was I endeavoured to 'fight my corner' on points of principle, not always with success, but openly with tenacity and I hope with integrity.

The role of 'Chairman' of any health authority will remain one of great challenge and great responsibility as 'champion of the people', differentiating between wants and needs, reconciling effective financial management with the hopes of professional staff for developing health care, and continuing a commitment to the overall philosophy of a National Health Service. The role of Chairman will surely bring to future holders of such posts the pleasure and fulfilment that it brought to colleagues and to me. My personal debt is great for the many happy years I have been privileged to spend in the Service.

Chapter 18
Postscript

Could there be life after St. Mary's?

Thankfully, there is!

The difficulty I had in separating myself from the Chairmanship of Paddington and North Kensington Health Authority was largely mitigated by the various other pursuits which overlapped and continued. I was succeeded by Michael Hatfield, whose courtesy and friendship in inviting me to various social occasions did much to lessen the inevitable regrets I felt in leaving - another bereavement like that of leaving office in Cornwall. Being human, there are naturally occasions in matters at a national level, when I should still like to exert the influence which the position of Chairman allows.

My second term of office with the Medical Research Council still had two years to run when I left St. Mary's. My appointment with the Industrial Tribunals continued, as did my great interest in the Magistracy. In 1987 I was appointed to the Lambeth, Southwark and Lewisham Family Practitioner Committee which in 1990 became the Family Health Services Authority, and there I continue to serve as Vice-Chairman. Just as there

were differences both in kind and in degree between the needs of patients in Cornwall and in
Paddington so there are cultural and other differences between Paddington and Lambeth.
What is appropriate to one may not be so in the
other. But, once more I feel privileged to continue
to work in the health service, to assist those who
are working in a deprived inner city area, and to
play a part - albeit small - in the further history of
the NHS.

   In 1988 I joined a small management consultancy
firm and consequently have had new opportunities to visit Health Authorities in widely separated parts of the country. In addition, I have
made many good friends. Reflecting on my good
fortune in committing myself professionally and
without reservation to a health service from the
position of a junior nurse to that of Chairman of
Health Authorities, through many changes on the
way, I have never regretted my commitment to
service which has given me so much more than I
could offer in return.

Appendix I

Extract from the report (1949) by E.R. Hargreaves, MA, MD, DPH

as reported in the British Medical Journal, April 15, 1950

POLIOMYELITIS IN CORNWALL IN 1949

During 1949, 110 cases of poliomyelitis occurred in Cornwall, giving an incidence of 0.3 per 1000 of the population, a little less than double the rate for England and Wales. The age distribution over the country as a whole was normal - namely, approximately one-third under school age, one-third 5 - 14, and one-third 15 and over. Distribution of the first 100 cases is shown in Figure 1.

It will be noted that there were four main centres of infection in the County, Camborne-Redruth, Penzance, Fowey and Truro. It is interesting to compare this distribution with that of 1947 and to note that areas most affected in that year were relatively free of the disease in 1949.

The Camborne-Redruth outbreak was the first in the County; indeed, other than Newhaven, it was the first group of cases in the country. On June 21 three cases of paralysis were notified in Illogan, a village some four miles from Redruth. During the subsequent two months 21 further cases occurred in the Camborne-Redruth Urban District and one at Truro School. An interesting feature of this small outbreak was the age group affected, 56% being under 5 years old.

The outbreak was for some time confined to the village of Illogan and it seemed certain that the source of infection was close at hand. Of the initial three cases, two were pupils at the Illogan Infants' School and the other, a child of three, had an elder sister there. Careful investigation of the food supply and hygiene of the school together with the movements of staff and pupils failed to uncover any possible origin of the outbreak. Consideration was given to the possibility of the importation of the virus from outside, but no visitors had stayed in any of the affected houses during the previous six weeks, nor had the occupants been away on holiday. Two old cases of poliomyelitis were known to be present in the district but as it was two years since they contracted the disease the possibility of their still carrying the virus seemed remote.

Five more cases occurred in Illogan, all intimately connected with the school, four being pupils; the fifth, a child of 2 1/2 had a brother at the school.

From Illogan the disease spread to Camborne and Redruth, Truro and St. Day. When peripheral spreading occurs it is usually fairly easy to trace the origin of the first case. In Redruth, for instance, a case was notified on June 29, and on June 30 two boys in an adjoining house developed paralysis. The two families had gone by bus to Portreath beach on June 20 and again on June 21. The bus route is through Illogan, and many children from the village had joined the bus.

The first case in Camborne was admitted to the Isolation Hospital on July 8. The patient was a cousin of an Illogan case, and his aunt, in spite of warnings, had visited his home on two occaisons, the last being eight days previously.

One solitary case was reported from Truro School; the boy developed paralysis on July 12, the infection being possibly contracted on June 25, when he went to a large religious meeting at Gwennap Pit, near St. Day and subsequently spent the evening in Redruth.

Two cases occurred in St. Day; both had had indirect contact with Illogan. At Fowey the outbreak started with a burst at the beginning of August, when five children developed paralytic poliomyelitis within 48 hours of one another. Again it was the pre-school children that suffered, four of the five cases being under 5 years of age. The area MOH investigated this outbreak in great detail but could find no common factor. The water supply was extremely low at the time, but reports proved satisfactory. The boiling of water and milk was advocated.

The stage seemed set for a serious outbreak, but only three more cases occurred in the town, all developing paralysis two weeks later. One was an indirect contact through her sister with a previous case. The interval was 16 days, which allowed time for the virus to become established in the sister although she developed no symptoms suggestiive of abortive poliomyelitis. The other two cases were close contacts, both working in the local chemist's shop.

It is fascinating, but often extremely difficult, to trace the origin of outbreaks such as occurred at Fowey. One felt that some connexion with the Camborne-Redruth cases probably existed and searched accordingly; but in mid-August a letter from Dr. A.M. McFarlan, of Cambridge, told of a clerk from Cambridge and her fiance who visited Polruan for their holiday on July 24, leaving again on August 9. While there the son of the hotel proprietor was ill for two days with symptoms suggestive of abortive poliomyelitis, and within a few dys of returning to their homes - the girl to Cambridge, her fiance to Scunthorpe - both these visitors developed paralytic poliomyelitis.

Polruan, the"'Penpoodle' of Sir Arthur Quiller-Couch's Troy Town, is in reality a part of Fowey, being separated from the main portion of the town by the River Fowey. A visit unearthed the history of two further visitors to Polruan who developed poliomyelitis after returning home, the earliest date being June 27, six weeks before the onset of the Fowey cases and approximately the same date as the beginning of the Illogan outbreak, some 40 miles away.

A violent focus of infection appeared in the city of Truro (population 12,950) at the beginning of September. Two cases of paralysis were reported on September 11, and in the subsequent 10 days 12 more patients were admitted to the County Isolation Hospital. In all, some 20 cases occurred in Truro and a further seven in the surrounding villages. Paralysis was severe, particularly in early cases, four of which proved fatal.

Figure 1: map of Cornwall

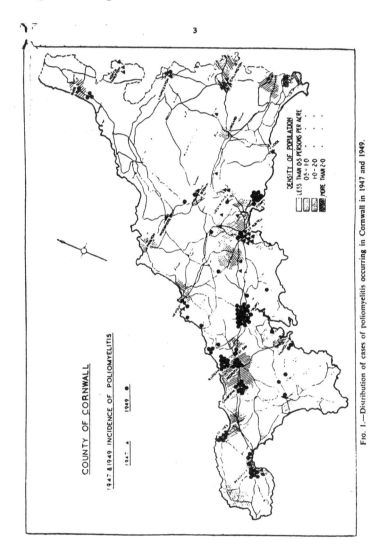

FIG. 1.—Distribution of cases of poliomyelitis occurring in Cornwall in 1947 and 1949.

Appendix II

Transcript of letter addressed to Mr. M. Lillywhite, Private
Secretary, Private Office to the Minister of State for Health
and Social Security, Alexander Fleming House, Elephant &
Castle, London, SEl 6BY

17th October 1975
Dear Mr. Lillywhite,
              Optimum Use of Resources
You will recall that when we met on Wednesday, 1st October,
you indicated that it would be helpful if I were to let you have,
in broad outline, some account of the apparently insuperable
difficulties in Cornwall due to an acknowledged shortfall of
resources (as seen at the time) and the manner in which,
through Operational Research, we are endeavouring to provide a safe and efficient service.

I have looked through the voluminous files of correspond-
ence and documents and have selected those which would
seem to be of particular significance.

You will note the acknowledged shortfall of beds (Page 1 -
Appendix I) and you will note the strict terms of reference,
whereby the Study must relate to optimum use of existing
resources (Page 2 - Appendix 2).

If I were to attempt to describe the chaotic state of the
hospital service prior to the presence of the OR Team, you
would probably think it exaggerated but I assure you that the
service existed in an atmosphere of crisis, heightened tension
in medical (consultant and junior) staff, and constant disen-
chantment and high wastage of nursing staff. Patients were
being moved from ward to ward and hospital to hospital like
yo-yos, sometimes as much as seven times in one short stay
and often in the night. Frequently all admissions other than
acute emergencies had to be refused throughout the clinical

area, patients sent for, were returned home, with all the consequent distress and anxiety, not to say fury, of patients and their relatives.

As a result of the presence of the OR Team and the Study undertaken, there is now a recognised procedure whereby impending crises in the bed state are recognised and dealt with (Appendix 4), an information room is in operation, studies have been made of the Medical and Surgical (bed) resources and theatre time (Appendices 5 and 6), and of problems relating to head injuries and self-administered poisonings (Appendix 7).

Despite an influenza epidemic, an increasing ratio of over 65s to the total population with consequent demands on services, the usual enormous influx of holiday population and with no additional capital resources other than 20 medical beds created at Tehidy in 1973, the Service managed without the need to impose a red alert throughout the spring, summer and autumn 1975.

The Study in itself has been of inestimable value in demonstrating alternatives, in stimulating discussion and in acting as a catalyst as between consultants and their G.P. colleagues, but above all as a means whereby a change of emphasis has been achieved so that the criteria for an efficient service is no longer restricted to the provision of beds as being the sole meaningful measurement. A very important additional benefit has accrued through enhanced job satisfaction for nursing staff, resulting from and in better patient care, decreasing wastage in nurse training (no vacancies in the School of Nursing until 1977) and above all a decrease in the number of complaints from patients and their relatives within this particular context.

The OR Team in consultation with medical staff are in process of preparing an admissions policy for RCH (Treliske) (Appendix 8), this, I think, will be without precedence in the country and will be of great interest and importance to the Service. **Belinda Banham, Chairman**

10 documents appended: Memorandum, 8.4.1970: To South Western Regional Hospital Board; Letter from Junior Medical Staff: 31.12.1971; Letter to Sir John English: 6.1.1972; Commencement document: Proposals for an Operational Research Study of Cornwall H.M.C.; Letter to Mr. B. Holdaway, DHSS: 5.4.1973; Colour-coded Alert System Schedule for Information Room; Schedules: Medical Wards at Treliske, and Surgical Wards at Treliske, September 1974-March 1975; Statistics: Head Injuries and Self-Administered Poisoning; Two documents: a) Admissions Policy for General Surgical Wards, July 1975 and b) Towards a Medical Admissions Policy, July 1975. [Documents not included here for reasons of space.]

Extract from paper delivered in Paris, 1975.

The use of operational research in resource allocation in the Cornwall area

B.Banham, Cornwall Area Health Authority, Truro, U.K.
C.E.R. Tristem, Department of Health & Social Security, London, U.K.

After a period of assessment, three aspects of the problem were studied: (1) the reallocation of beds between specialities at the central hospital and peripheral hospitals, (2) the development of admission stragies and (3) the monitoring of the effects of any changes in these areas. Study of the reallocation of beds led to the consideration of communication problems between the central and peripheral hospitals. An information room was opened at Treliske during a trial period of six months to act as a bed bureau for the area. It is working well.

Examination of the requirements of any admission policy to the central hospitals enforced the view that a monitoring system for changes is necessary. Effort was therefore concentrated on developing a system of information collection on patient flows (from HAA returns) and resource usage (from hospital data).

A monthly analysis of this data has helped to identify bottlenecks, and create discussion of how these might be removed or alternatively to see how admissions strategies might be modified to eliminate intolerable overloading of resources.

1.Introduction

Early in December 1973 the OR team at DHSS were asked to see if they could help with the problem of over stretched resources in the Cornwall Area Health Authority. The provision of hospital facilities in this area comprised a District General Hospital (370 beds) of which there were two units separated by one and a half miles. RCH(City) contained Accident and Emergency, Orthopaedics, E.N.T., Ophthalmology and Paediatrics; RCH (Treliske) contained Acute Medicine and Surgery. All emergency admissions and waiting list cases in general medicine and general surgery tended to be directed to RCH (Treliske). The most obvious symptoms of the apparent lack of resources was excessive pressure on the District General Hospital in Truro where most of the acute health care for the area was taking place.

2. Investigation

The specific symptoms of pressure which became apparent to the OR team early on, was the bed occupancy levels at the two central hospitals; one of them, Treliske, was frequently running at 105 per cent occupancy and consequently all admissions from the waiting lists were frequently suspended. This was accompanied by an under utilization of the four peripheral hospitals, where occupancies, on occasions were as low as 50 per cent. The result of high occupancy at the centre was increased length of surgical waiting lists and of waiting time, a lowering of staff morale which in turn led to increased wastage particularly in nursing staff. There were other symptoms of pressure including a high number of transfers of patients from one ward in hospitals to other wards as well as protest meetings of medical and nursing staff, and constant complaints from patients and their relatives.

At first the general feeling of the staff was that the problem of the two hospitals at the AHA could only be solved by additional resources in the form of beds. This was not an option open to the consideration by the OR team but it took some time to convince senior consultants and nurses that the solution must result from re-organisation and re-allocation of existing resources.

Initially two ways were recognised by which current overloading of the District General Hospital might be alleviated. One was by control of admissions and discharges (the development of an admission policy) the other by more intensive utilization of the beds and other facilities in the smaller hospitals outside Truro which form part of the total resources available in Cornwall. However, it was recognised early on, that whatever improvement might be made in the utilisation of resources in the peripheral hospitals a significant reduction in the load on the main hospitals in Truro was unlikely to accrue from this source alone. It therefore followed that some patient currently being treated in hospital would need to be cared for either wholly in the community or by different combinations of community and hospital care. For this reason community physicians (then called medical officer of health) and family practitioners (then called general practitioners) were co-opted onto the team. This in itself had a salutory effect because it emphasized the continuing nature of the general practitioners caring role as contrasted with the incident based function performed by the hospital services.

3. Intensive utilization of beds and other facilities
3.1 Reallocation of beds

As described above it had been observed that the resources of the peripheral hospitals were not being utilized at the same lvel of intensity as those in the centre. The first attempt to improve the level of usage was directed at redeploying the specialties to different hospitals within the area. Several alternative patterns of allocation of hospital beds to specialties were examined. This was a complex process requiring much consultation since there existed a large number of constraints as to the location of specialties in peripheral hospitals. Eventually certain recommendations were made which would allow a more rational use of the peripheral hospitals and some of these are being adopted.

3.2 The information room

At the same time as the work on the reallocation of beds was being carried out another method of making better use of the peripheral facilities was also being explored. This was to set up an information room at the central hospital in the area with a primary duty to maintain, twice daily, information on the bed states of all hospitals in the area. This allowed the consultants to transfer patients from the District General Hospital to the peripheral hospitals when it was felt to be medically acceptable and/or when the pressure on beds in the District General Hospital had reached too high a level. The result of the introduction of the information room was to increase significantly the occupancy of the peripheral hospitals. This initially had the effect of reducing occupancy levels at the centre. The success of the information room in achieving better resource utilisation meant that the implementation of the study on reallocation of beds to specialties became less urgent. Some of the suggestions, however, have benefits in their own right and while only one major option has as yet been adopted, the elimination of further bed reallocation as a major option has forced the hospital staff to consider realistic alternatives.

4. Resource control and monitoring at hospital level (not reprinted here for reasons of space)

5. The capacity of the operating theatres

By the time the studies on reallocation of beds and the information room had been completed, the system of problem defining, information gathering, evaluation and action as described above was in full operation. The system was monitoring a variety of factors and the principal users of resources (the surgeons and physicians) started holding regular meetings at which the analysis of information was discussed. The result of this was to detect that several resources other than beds were acting as constraints upon the efficient running of hospitals. The first of those examined was operating theatres. Consideration was given to the workload on the theatres, the factors influencing the capacity of the theatres, e.g. staff, demands on theatre time (such as theatre maintenance, cleaning, etc.) the capacity of central sterile supply to provide sterile instruments, theatre porters, etc. The critical resources appeared to be theatre nurses, CSSD and possibly portering. Recommendations to reduce these constraints and allow greater theatre capacity were made accordingly and extra nursing staff were trained and appointed. A time limit was placed on duration of operating lists (excluding unforseen emergencies).

6. Towards a medical admissions policy

The running of the information/intelligence system in conjunction with the information room ensures a continued management of the hospitals' resources, but one way of anticipating problems is to institute an admissions and discharge policy. It was envisaged that the information room could be developed by the appointment of an admissions officer who would, with the aid of a consultant where necessary decide on the admission or otherwise of patients referred to the hospitals and if admitted, to which hospital. No case would be refused admission without prior agreement of the consultant.

6.1 Criteria for allocating patients

Given the 'admissions officer' as envisaged above, equipped with up-to-date bed state information, it is necessary to provide him with adequate rules for allocating admissions between the hospitals. It seemed likely that referrals would be grouped according to age, sex, diagnosis and home circumstances so that guidelines of the following types could be set up (there may be others):

(i) Patients in category W go to hospital A as first choice. If no beds are available try hospital B.

(ii) Patients in category X go to hospital A. If no beds are available (or if this admission will create a congested bed state) contact hospital A and ask if any additional beds could be cleared.

(iii) Patients in category Y are shared as evenly as possible between hospitals A and C.

(iv) Patients in category Z are not normally admitted.

Much of this has now been done, and some of these rules were determined by the location of laboratories and consultant specialties. Other criteria were determined by discussion between the consultant involved. The success of the above depends, in part, on how far the admissions officer is able to take over the allocation of patients without needing to refer this decision to consultants, thus the more cases covered by allocation rules which have been agreed with all the physicians concerned, the more effective the scheme will be.

6.2 Monitoring the admissions policy

The admissions and discharge policy will be maintained by the information/intelligence system and modified in the light of any difficulties so identified. A similar policy for the surgical specialties is currently being discussed.

7. The results of the OR work [at date of Report, 1976]

a. Whilst throughput for the hospitals group has increased the occupancy in the District General Hospital has been much reduced. It now averages the target level of 85-90 per cent.

The average occupancy of RCH (Treliske) is now in the region of 85 per cent.

b. The above has had the effect of relieving much of the pressure on the nursing staff with a consequent improvement in morale and wastage rates.

c. The number of inter-ward transfers has been reduced.

d. Despite the recent 'work to contract' on the part of consultants and junior medical staff, surgical waiting lists which stood at 2,200 in December, 1973, are currently at 1,600; during this period an extra surgeon was appointed. However, the appointment of an additional surgeon represents only one factor in an improved situation. Prior to the installation of the information room and the information/intelligence system, initially beds, subsequently nurses and theatre time were the critical resources. It is a combination of the additional appointment and the OR work done on alleviating pressure on resources that has effected a reduction in the waiting lists.

e. There have been no occasions upon which it has been necessary to suspend admissions from the waiting lists since the start of the study.

f. Complaints from members of the staff, patients and their relatives have fallen dramatically.

Acknowledgement: The Authors wish to thank the medical and nursing staff in Cornwall and the National Coal Board OR Group for their very significant contribution to the work this paper describes.

Index